PRAISE FOR *DR. LANI'S NO-NONSENSE SUN HEALTH GUIDE*

"Contrary to what you've been told, sun exposure is absolutely crucial to vibrant health. But you have to know how to get the right dose at the right time, without harming the skin. *Dr. Lani's No- Non-sense Sun Health Guide* is full of life-saving information that everyone needs to know. I highly recommend this book for everyone!"

—Christiane Northrup, MD *New York Times bestselling* author of *The Wisdom of Menopause and Goddesses Never Age.*

"Slip, slap, slop? Not so fast. Thankfully, Dr. Lani Simpson untangles our complicated relationship with the sun, and offers an enlightened approach to vitamin D supplementation. On a topic in which misleading information abounds, Dr. Lani's thoughtful advice shines through."

—Kate Rhéaume, N.D. Author of *Vitamin K2 and the Calcium Paradox: How a Little - Known Vitamin Could Save Your Life*

"*Dr. Lani's No-Nonsense Sun Health Guide* provides not only a wealth of facts about vitamin D and its relationship to bone and overall health, but it will help you understand UV radiation, skin cancer, sunscreen products, and the difference between supplemental vitamin D, and that derived from the skin's exposure to the sun. I highly recommend this book!"

—R. Keith McCormick, DC, author of *The Whole-Body Approach to Osteoporosis*, founder of OsteoNaturals, ten-time world championship competitor, and U.S. Olympian.

"Vitamin D and safe sun exposure are vital to our health. Unfortunately, many doctors and patients do not understand how to utilize these for optimal health. In this timely and important book, Dr. Lani Simpson provides a clear and detailed approach that we can all benefit from."

—Sunjya Schweig, MD CEO and Co-director California Center for Functional Medicine

Dr. Lani has done it again! Another well-written No-Nonsense guide book to understanding the nuances and importance of how our body transforms Vitamin D for our bones and our overall health, the best lab to measure vitamin D and the acceptable "D" range. Diving deeply into the differences of sunscreen vs sunblock, SPF, the best sun-protecting clothing, and how to safely sun-worship with a simple chart as a guide, offers crucial, easy-to-follow tips that keeps the reader engaged. As with *Dr. Lani's No-Nonsense Bone Health Guide*, I will be bringing No-Nonsense Sun Health Guide to my community.

—Irma Jennings, INHC Holistic Bone Coach Food4HealthyBones.com

"I highly recommend this book on an important subject. Dr. Lani provides expert advice and information in a very readable format. You will learn a great deal that may surprise you and perhaps even transform your relationship to the sun, sunscreens and vitamin D. There are pearls for the both general folks and health professionals."

—Judy Lane, NP, MS Director of Women's Health at the Preventive Medical Center of Marin, Inc. and Director of Women's Health Programs at the EarthRose Institute.

DR. LANI'S

No-Nonsense
Sun Health Guide

The Truth About
Vitamin D, Sensible Sun Exposure,
Sunscreens, *and* Skin Cancer

Dr. Lani Simpson, DC, CCD

TURNER PUBLISHING COMPANY

Turner Publishing Company
Nashville, Tennessee
New York, New York
www.turnerpublishing.com

The information contained in this book is based upon the research and personal and professional experiences of the author. It is not intended as a substitute for consulting with your physician or other healthcare provider. Any attempt to diagnose and treat an illness should be done under the direction of a healthcare professional.

The publisher does not advocate the use of any particular healthcare protocol but believes the information in this book should be available to the public. The publisher and author are not responsible for any adverse effects or consequences resulting from the use of the suggestions, preparations, or procedures discussed in this book. Should the reader have any questions concerning the appropriateness of any procedures or preparation mentioned, the author and the publisher strongly suggest consulting a professional healthcare advisor.

Library of Congress Cataloging-in-Publication Data
Names: Simpson, Lani, author.
Title: Dr. Lani's no-nonsense sun health guide : the truth about; vitamin D, sensible sun exposure, sunscreens, and skin cancer.
Other titles: No-nonsense sun health guide
Description: Nashville : Turner Publishing Company, 2019. |
Identifiers: LCCN 2018049259 (print) | LCCN 2018051820 (ebook) | ISBN 9781684423040 (ebook) | ISBN 9781684423026 (pbk.) | ISBN 9781684423033 (hardcover)
Subjects: LCSH: Sunshine--Therapeutic use. | Sunshine--Health aspects. | Health behavior.
Classification: LCC RM843 (ebook) | LCC RM843 .S56 2019 (print) | DDC 613/.193--dc23
LC record available at https://lccn.loc.gov/2018049259

Cover design: Maddie Cothren
Book design: Tim Holtz

Printed in the United States of America

10 9 8 7 6 5 4 3 2 1

For my beloved partner in life, Audrey Martin. Without your generosity, love and support this book would never have seen the light of day.

And for Sam Martin, whom I love and deeply respect.

Contents

Foreword

Over the past ten years, I have enjoyed a professionally collaborative and warm personal friendship with Dr. Lani Simpson. When I first started reading the book, I did not expect not to be able to put it down. I learned so much from this book and thoroughly enjoyed Dr. Simpson's accessible writing style. Chapter 1 immediately engaged me, as I read about the role of the sun in different cultures in the ancient world, ranging from worshipping it (the Egyptians) to avoiding it (the Greeks). It also set the nuanced tone for the entire book, explaining the value of the sun in producing vitamin D while recognizing the risks of burns and cancer.

Dr. Lani's No Nonsense Sun Health Guide lives up to its name, No-nonsense. It is refreshing to read a more balanced point of view regarding sun exposure. Some doctors recommend sun avoidance completely while others promote sun exposure. Dr. Simpson's recommendation regarding a mindful relationship with the sun is very important as she points out, "Don't Get Burned", warning us against intense sun exposure, as well as chronic sun exposure without the use of practical measures to protect the skin.

Although she has sustained over 20 skin cancers and is at high risk of developing melanoma, she still exposes her skin to mindful and limited sunlight to make some of her vitamin D. Dr. Simpson discusses pre-cancers, skin cancer types, diagnosis, and treatment options including Western Medicine. She also offers her opinion regarding alternative treatments for skin cancers and nutrition for healthy skin and supplements that may be beneficial for reducing future skin cancers.

Vitamin D is another hot topic with a wide range of opinions about the optimal dose for good health. Vitamin D in its active form is one of the most powerful hormones in the body. Vitamin D deficiency is common in the Northern hemisphere and supplementation for the vast majority of people is important for their well-being. Dr. Simpson explains how important it is not to take too much vitamin D and to make sure that your serum calcium is not high enough to lead to other health issues.

When I read the chapter on sunscreens, I ran to my cabinet to check the ingredients in my products. Unfortunately, the products I have been using are not safe for me nor for the environment. There is a handy section on ingredients to avoid and the best ones to use.

The section on skin cancer provided a good understanding of the types of skin cancer and the importance of checking your own skin for possible skin cancers. Her section on skin examination and treatment options for skin cancers are valuable additions. In addition, she shares her own experiences regarding incorrect skin cancer diagnosis and treatment options.

In the final chapter on Circadian Rhythms she delves into the importance of light itself to set our internal clock and to be in sync with the planet on which we live. Sleep disorders are common, especially in women and especially as we age. The practical advice in this chapter will help many who have sleep issues.

Dr. Lani's No Nonsense Sun Health Guide is full of useful information and practical advice. It even included a detailed description of the best clothes and hats and sunglasses to minimize sun exposure! And what I found particularly appealing was that her explanations and advice were thoroughly researched, summarizing studies that support different opinions regarding several of the subjects she discussed, and then providing her own well-thought-out opinions and recommendations. All in all, Dr. Simpson has written a well-researched and highly accessible guide for anyone interested in how to incorporate safe sun exposure into their life in order to optimize their vitamin D levels without triggering skin cancer or getting burned.

Jennifer Schneider M.D., Ph.D. is a physician specializing in Internal Medicine, Addiction Medicine, and Pain Medicine. Dr. Schneider is the author of 13 books and multiple medical articles. She has a particular interest in bone health and osteoporosis after sustaining an atypical femur fracture (AFF) as a result of prolonged bisphosphonate treatment. She now helps patients who have sustained such fractures.

Acknowledgments

I wish to thank the following people, whose expertise and support—both technical and emotional—have made this book possible. Each of you has had a significant impact on my work over the years, and I thank you deeply.

Gwen Simpson and Jack Simpson, RIP and the rest of the Simpson clan. Sigrid Herr and Hadas Rin, and Jeremy Nash. Cheryl Edwards for your patience in editing this book with me and your kind support. Paci, Larry, and Nina Goldman; Bernie and Sadie Horowitz; Germaine Deluca; Fran; Brad and Karen Martin; Ron Martin and Grandma Eve who still live in our hearts, and the rest of the Chicago tribe. To Malgosia Treter-Bogatski for your amazing generosity, support and editing suggestions. Jean Kaufman and Terri Rubinstein for your exceptional kindness and support; Carole Goldberg; Sheryl Green; Tuyet Cong-Ton-Nu for your peaceful presence and wisdom; Judy Lane, NP for your extraordinary knowledge; Mary Clair Blakeman who started this book journey with me many years ago; Lizzy Steger; Adela Lopez, Bonnie Halpern and to Ann and Lisa for our years of friendship. Dr. Warren Dotz, whose skill as a dermatologist for which I will always be indebted. Dr. Jennifer Schneider for her endless knowledge, collaboration and support. To my Bone Health Master Class and to our amazing Facebook group: Osteoporosis—Myths and Facts.

Wilbur Hot Springs, where much of this book was written. To the amazing crew: I am deeply saddened by the loss of the great hotel by fire, but the memories and the land will live forever!

Introduction

My first encounter with skin cancer involved outpatient surgery to remove a small growth from my forearm. Later another carcinoma was excised from my back. Then, soon after my third skin cancer diagnosis in 1999, I participated in a five-day silent retreat at Spirit Rock, a meditation center in northern California. It was winter, and after ten straight days of wind and rain, the sun emerged into the background of a perfectly blue sky.

To celebrate this gift and to shake out the days of sitting and struggling with a very active mind, I set out for an afternoon hike. The air was clean, fresh, and unusually warm, allowing me a taste of early spring. After climbing several steep hills, I found a sweet resting spot on a swatch of damp grass. I wanted to feel the sun on my skin, but, because I had become accustomed to always wearing clothing that provided a safe barrier against the penetrating ultraviolet rays, I hesitated. Would a few glorious minutes basking in the sun really be harmful, or could it actually be healthy for me? The warmth was irresistible; I removed my sun hat and long-sleeved shirt. As the heat warmed my body, tears welled up, and as they streamed down my face, my fear melted. The days of meditation fully opened me to this moment with the sun, my old friend. Thus, I began a renewed, conscious relationship with our world's source of light and life.

In my early years, my relationship with the sun was anything but conscious. As a child, I lived in the sun's rays, water-skiing every summer and playing outside whenever possible. My tanned skin was dark, thanks to Portuguese ancestry, but I am Scottish and Irish, too, which makes me especially susceptible to burning until a tan is established. Every year I suffered several second-degree burns with large blisters—one so severe that for two days I couldn't walk without help and almost landed in the hospital.

In my teens, I sunbathed regularly in my backyard. To make sure my tan was even, I wrapped aluminum foil over cardboard to reflect the sun onto the sides of my body, thereby maximizing my likelihood of acquiring an agonizing sunburn. And although my mother thought she was helping, she made matters worse by basting my blistered skin with butter, which actually increased the damage. Every year, sunburns and peeling layers of dead skin were part of my summer experience. My mother and I added additional skin trauma by using dermatologist-recommended, UVB-emitting sunlamps to create sunburns on our faces, which was, at one time, considered a remedy for acne. Of course, we wanted that "healthy glow" look as well. Looking back, I wonder if we suffered some form of amnesia, as we repeated this yearly ritual over and over again.

In my early forties, I was diagnosed with borderline osteoporosis, and the diagnosis frightened me to my core. At that time, I attributed my low bone mass to never having developed good bone-building habits as a teenager. An estimated 80 to 90 percent of peak bone mass is acquired by age eighteen in girls and by age twenty in boys, which makes youth the best time to "invest" in one's bone health. During my adolescence, I had a poor diet, didn't exercise, and smoked a pack of cigarettes daily. So, having porous bones seemed a likely consequence of those poor health habits during my teen years. However, despite my mid-life efforts to build bone through a better diet and exercise regimen (and without ingesting commonly prescribed osteoporosis drugs), I continued to lose density.

Ten years later, a blood test revealed that I had vitamin D deficiency. *What? I had a vitamin D deficiency while living in California?* The answer was simple: I live near the ocean, and the fog is often thick during summer months, which is just when we should be building up our stores of vitamin D for the winter. In addition, I bought into the notion that the sun was to be avoided at all times, especially midday, which is exactly when the particular ray that produces vitamin D is the strongest.

Two other health conditions emerged in my forties that I now relate, in part, to vitamin D deficiency: hypothyroidism and deep muscular and bone pain in both hips. The bilateral hip pain was so severe that I couldn't get a good night's sleep; the mere weight of my small body on a mattress would cause teeth-clenching episodes that worsened even though I practiced yoga and had chiropractic care and massage treatment. As it turns out, vitamin D deficiency can cause both muscle and bone pain, and the thyroid relies on vitamin D to function properly. These revelations awakened me to the breadth of the functioning of vitamin D in the body—and provided my first indication that vitamin D is not merely a vitamin but is actually a type of hormone. It is, in fact, one of the most powerful hormones in the body. Only after I increased my vitamin D levels significantly, in my early fifties, did my hip pain finally resolve.

So, while I fried in the sun in my early years, I did not get enough sun in adulthood! For my own health, I needed to unravel the plethora of research papers and opinions from experts in the fields of vitamin D, osteoporosis, and skin cancer. As one research article led to another, and I delved ever deeper, I realized how little of the fast-expanding body of knowledge about the sun's vital role in our health maintenance was available in an accessible and understandable format. So, what started out as a thirty-page pamphlet turned into this book, *Dr. Lani's No-Nonsense Sun Health Guide*. Given the ramifications

> ". . . while I fried in the sun in my early years, I did not get enough sun in adulthood!"

of either too much or too little sunshine, my recommendations here are based on research and, at times, good old common sense.

Excessive sun exposure can indeed increase skin cancer risk, yet the sun is essential for our health and well-being. The sunshine vitamin is a key ingredient for crucial bodily functions, including supporting bone growth as well as the nervous and immune systems. Vitamin D deficiency has been implicated in a wide range of disease processes including diabetes, multiple sclerosis, heart disease, depression, leukemia, eczema, many forms of cancer, and a host of additional ailments discussed further in forthcoming chapters of this book. And the added benefit of sunlight itself is crucial in maintaining a healthy mental status, as well as stimulating hormones necessary for a good night's sleep.

Today, informed and aware of the benefits and risks of sun exposure, I sunbathe cautiously in order to produce some natural vitamin D, knowing that the sun can both heal and harm. I am hardly wanton regarding my time in the sun; in fact, quite the opposite, I am fully present and conscious of exactly how much exposure I receive. With this book, I offer a practical guide for a relationship with the sun—one devoid of fear yet imbued with cautious awareness.

I'll also provide you information about how sun exposure can produce vitamin D, as well as a frank discussion about the risks of skin cancer. In addition, this book covers concerns about sunscreens. We've been told to slather up with sunscreen products, but—surprise—there's estrogen in that sunscreen! Studies have confirmed that many of the active chemical ingredients in sunscreen products exhibit hormonal activity.

I have melded my concerns about these chemicals, and I offer advice on the best ingredients to look for—for you and your family. As well, a section of this book is devoted to a list of chemicals that consumers need to be aware of and avoid.

My journey, which started out as a quest to improve my own health, led me to question and learn what the body needs for optimal functioning. In that pursuit, I discovered that the sun, while often a source of joy and pleasure, also plays a vitally important and central role for our overall health. Here I share with you what I have learned in the hope that your life, too, is enhanced with sunlight, more joy, and better health.

Chapter 1

The Sun: Friend or Foe?

Since time began, we have alternately worshipped and feared the sun. In the ancient world, Egyptians revered the sun god, Ra. The Greeks, however, warned their children to avoid the fate of Icarus, the mythical boy who plunged to his death when he flew too close to the sun with his waxen wings. Sun worship has defined religious practices. The sun is most often depicted as the male principal, balanced by the female aspect in the form of the moon, or occasionally the earth. In all such theologies, the sun represents the giver of life.

Egyptian kings believed they descended from Ra, the sun god. Similarly, in the ancient Hindu religion, Surya, a primary deity, represents the sun. God manifesting as the sun is found in Africa's Liza, the Celts' Lugh, the Polynesian Maui, the Roman and Greeks' Apollo, the Pueblo Indians' Tawa, and the Inca's Inti. One of the few female representations of the sun, Amaterasu, is found in Japanese worship; she was the Great Sun Goddess of Japan and queen of all the Kami, representing all the forces inherent in nature. The hearts of Jesus and of the Virgin Mary are often represented by a sun symbol in early Christian paintings.

Chakra, the Sanskrit word meaning "energy center," describes seven spots in the body that correspond to certain areas along the spine and head. The heart chakra located in the center of the chest symbolizes the sun and the high emotional center and guardian of the solar system. At the break of dawn, Yogis gather along the banks of the Ganges River to assume with unimaginable physical suppleness the sun salutations, a series of yoga postures by which they honor the new day.

The oldest known monuments—such as Stonehenge, the Druids' sophisticated structure in Great Britain, as well as the North American Indians' Bighorn Medicine Wheel in Wyoming and the temples of the Maya in Central America—were all places of worship as well as complex instruments by which time and the seasons were charted, with astonishing accuracy. The concept of the twenty-four-hour day originates with Egyptians' sun worship. To this day, the precision and sophistication of the ancient mathematicians, astronomers, and builders—without the technology we take for granted—is all but unimaginable.

Across time, right up to and including the popular culture of this century and the last, the sun has inspired great creativity, enlightening dance, the visual arts, and music, including all-time hits such as The Beatles' "Here Comes the Sun" and "Good Day Sunshine," as well as the 5th Dimension's "Let the Sunshine In," and Stevie Wonder's, "You Are the Sunshine of My Life." Classical composers, too, wrote pieces that radiated light, including Michel-Richard De Lalande's *Music for the Sun King* and Edvard Grieg's "Morning." The Indian ragas are based on time of day and the sun's position in the sky. The Sun Dance was the most spectacular and important religious ceremony of the Plains Indians of North America. Invoking the sun in all art forms, including dance and song, conveys warmth, brightness, and a general sense of well-being. Such ritualistic representations remind us that the sun is both pleasurable and essential for the health of body and mind, when experienced mindfully and in moderation.

In the twenty-first century, these positive and negative aspects of the sun continue to manifest. On the one hand, we desire the benefits of solar energy, but on the other, we worry about the impact of global warming.

Our individual health concerns should also include the power of the sun to harm and to heal. We are constantly told to cover up with hats, slather on sunscreen, and stay out of the sun to avoid the risk of skin cancer, a disease that has been on the rise for the past several decades. Yet, simultaneously, we hear that we need more sunshine to create vitamin D, a beneficial substance that can actually help prevent numerous forms of cancer as well as osteoporosis. Unfortunately, so many of us are working indoors or covering up because of skin cancer fears that an estimated one billion people worldwide suffer from vitamin D deficiency. In fact, the problem has reached such a point that epidemiologists are reporting a global resurgence of rickets, a serious condition triggered by an extreme lack of vitamin D that stunts children's growth, causes bowed legs, and negatively impacts brain development—and most people assumed this disease was conquered in the 1930s in the United States.

How can we sort out these conflicting messages? Is there a safe middle ground between embracing the sun as a benevolent friend or rejecting it as a dangerous foe? Most importantly, for the purposes of this book, how do we tap into the sun's energy for the vitamin D we want—without triggering the skin cancer that we don't want? And what do we do when we can't rely on the sun alone for all of the vitamin D we need?

By the time you finish this book, you will know the answers to those questions. You will learn when, where, and how the majority of people can expose themselves to the sun's rays without getting burned. You will also find out:

- how vitamin D promotes an amazing array of health benefits beyond building strong bones;
- what distinguishes sun-produced vitamin D from vitamin D supplementation;
- how to test for and correct a vitamin D deficiency;
- how to enjoy sun exposure safely while reducing your risk of skin cancer;
- how to detect early skin changes that may be precancers or cancer;
- why it is crucial for most adults and children to supplement with vitamin D in addition to sensible sun exposure—especially in northern latitudes;
- why sunscreen chemicals can endanger your health—and how to select safe skin-care products for you and your family;
- how sunlight guides our circadian rhythms and promotes health;
- plus, more information to enable you to make informed decisions about your own health and that of your loved ones.

In addition, this book will help you understand the real dangers of unsafe sun exposure that can lead to skin damage and skin cancer, as well as the hype about vitamin D. Understandably there is a lot of excitement about all the newfound and potential benefits of vitamin D. The enthusiasm is justified because vitamin D comes as close to a "miracle" substance as any I have found. Nonetheless, it is not a cure-all, and throughout this book I will point out areas where I am concerned, such as the idea of people taking high doses of vitamin D without appropriate testing—a practice I advise against.

As you read this book, my hope is that you will be able to let go of unfounded fears and enjoy a healthy, mindful relationship with the sun. Ultimately, the sun is neither friend nor foe. Like the ocean, the sun is a force of nature, and its power to support or destroy life depends on how we respect that power and respond to it.

Creating a healthy relationship with the sun could start with appreciating the daily sunrise and sunset that we too often take for granted. Consider the enormity of the sun's impact on our lives. After all, the sun anchors the rotation of the planets and determines the growth of our food. And—even though it is located 93 million miles from the earth—the sun affects us intimately, down to the tiniest cells of our bodies.

This interaction—between the cells of our bodies and the rays of the sun—involves a complex interplay of natural and biological forces that subsequent chapters will focus on. This chapter is an overview to familiarize you with the basics of how the sun can heal, by creating vitamin D, and how it can hurt, by potentially triggering skin cancer. Let's begin with how we produce vitamin D from the sun.

On the Bright Side: Using the Sun to Make Vitamin D

The medical community has long acknowledged the important role vitamin D plays in helping the body absorb calcium and build bones. A burst of research in recent years has shown that vitamin D also plays a pivotal role in cancer and diabetes prevention and a slew of other health benefits that impact the heart, immune system, nervous system, and even brain chemistry. These reported research developments are not altogether surprising since vitamin D receptors are found throughout the body.

Further, vitamin D has multiple forms, and scientific discussions about the labels for the various forms of this substance are complicated. For simplicity's sake, I will be referring to vitamin D as the form that our skin makes from sun exposure and that we can get in supplements —that is, vitamin D3. Therefore, when you read the term *vitamin D* in this book, know that I am strictly talking about vitamin D3—except when it may be necessary to identify other forms of this substance. Although this may sound confusing, we will review in depth all of the different metabolites (forms) of vitamin D in Chapter 4.

Vitamin D: Vitamin or Hormone?

A vitamin is typically defined as a substance that the body requires but cannot produce itself. Yet this definition is not strictly true when applied to vitamin D because the human body is fully capable of synthesizing vitamin D through skin exposure to the sun's UVB rays. Researchers today know that vitamin D, in its active form, is a type of hormone. This concept was not fully understood during the 1920s, however, when rickets was rampant, and scientists discovered that cod liver oil was one cure for the disease. While investigating the elements of cod liver oil, researcher Elmer McCollum labeled one of these components "vitamin D" in a published paper. Although research about "vitamin D" is light years beyond that of McCollum's day, the name he gave to it stuck.

The fact that we still refer to it as a vitamin is not the only thing confusing about vitamin D. Vitamin D actually has dozens of metabolites (forms) with various names. For instance, the terms *calciol*, *calciferol*, and *cholecalciferol* are all used to label one form of vitamin D, that is, vitamin D3. There are also several forms of vitamin D supplements: pills or gel caps of vitamin D3 and vitamin D2 (ergocalciferol) are commonly seen on store shelves, and even cod liver oil contains a high level of D3. (I do not recommend cod liver oil or D2, a point that is addressed in Chapter 8.)

As noted previously, I will be using the term *vitamin D* in this book to refer to vitamin D3 (cholecalciferol). Where necessary, the specific name of other forms of vitamin D will be used. A complete discussion about the various forms of vitamin D and its role in bodily functions can be found in Chapter 4.

Important Note: Vitamin D Tests

The subject of vitamin-D testing is fully discussed in Chapter 6. You can refer to that chapter if you want to understand more about the results of this test if you've already taken it, or if you are planning on getting tested. What's important to note is that there are two lab tests that can be ordered for vitamin D: the 25-hydroxyvitamin D (25-D) test, and the 1,25-dihydroxyvitamin D3 (1,25-D) test. The correct method for evaluating vitamin D status is the 25-hydroxyvitamin D test. Sometimes, doctors will order the wrong test, so double-check which one is on the order form for the lab.

Before vitamin D can perform any of its life-enhancing functions, it has to enter the body in one of three ways:

- exposure to UVB rays
- supplementation
- diet

For now, we will focus on the UVB rays we absorb through sun exposure because it is the most natural way to obtain vitamin D. The illustration, "Turning the sun's rays into vitamin D," (Figure 1.1) provides a snapshot of this process.

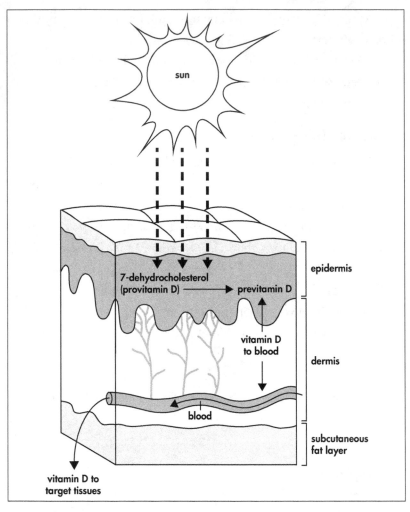

Turning the sun's rays into vitamin D (Figure 1.1)

As seen in the caption above, the sun emits UVB rays, which interact with a precursor to generate vitamin D3 (cholecalciferol). From the skin vitamin D3 is then transported to the liver where it undergoes another conversion to 25 (OH) D3. From the liver it is then transported to the kidneys for the final conversion to the active hormone vitamin D—1,25 (OH2) D3.

UVB vs. UVA?
Ultraviolet B rays (UVB—short wavelength).
Ultraviolet A rays (UVA—long wavelength).

Important Note: The sun's UVB rays—not its UVA rays—are the only ones that can produce vitamin D. So, if you are planning to sit in the sun to make vitamin D, it is crucial to know when and where UVB rays are available; otherwise, you're not only wasting your time but also needlessly exposing yourself to potentially damaging ultraviolet rays. In addition, sunscreen and sunscreen products absorb and block UVB rays effectively. For instance, skin-care products showing a Sun Protection Factor (SPF) 15 on the label will decrease skin penetration of UVB rays by 93 percent, thereby dramatically reducing the skin's ability to produce vitamin D. A full discussion of UV radiation is found in Chapter 2.

NOTE: The letters *A* and *B* following UV denote the name of the rays and nothing else. There is also a UVC ray that does not reach Earth, therefore is not important for our discussion.

Now that you have learned a little about how the sun can be a "friend," let's look at its role as a "foe" when excessive sun-exposure results in sunburn and cumulative damage.

Sun Exposure, the Downside: Skin Cancer and the Sun

One in five people will develop some form of skin cancer in their lifetimes. In recent years, an ongoing campaign has heightened public awareness about protecting the skin from the sun. In light of the constant barrage of media attention, there seem to be two extreme responses. One is to avoid sun–skin contact at all cost. The other is to ignore the warnings and allow sunburns to occur. Let me be clear: protecting the skin from the sun should be a daily assessment to avoid future skin cancers, and teaching children to be mindful and to respect the sun is a good practice.

Keep in mind that most skin cancers are easily treated when they are caught early. And even the most aggressive skin cancer, melanoma, is also treatable if caught early for those who are vigilant. In Chapter 9, you will learn how to identify questionable skin lesions. Clearly the word *cancer* sounds scary, and the first time I was diagnosed with a simple skin cancer on my arm, I was frightened into avoiding sun exposure. Over time, however, I learned that sensible sun exposure was far healthier than staying out of the sun completely.

It is important, then, to take skin cancer seriously; but at the same time, we also need to have a balanced approach when engaging with the sun. As you read this book, you will see that many factors are linked to skin cancer, including family history, genetic predisposition, age, and presence of excessive moles, as well as diet and cigarette smoking. Moderate, safe sun exposure has never been shown to cause skin cancer, except in people who have particularly strong hereditary factors. Excessive exposure to UV radiation from the sun, however, can contribute to the development of skin cancer in one of two ways:

1. Overexposure to the sun's UVB rays that result in sunburn. The more severe and frequent the burns, the higher the future risk of skin cancer, but even one burn increases your future risk of skin cancer. According to the Skin Cancer Foundation, "One blistering sunburn in childhood or adolescence more than doubles a person's chances of developing melanoma later in life. A person's risk for melanoma also doubles if he or she has had five or more sunburns at any age."

2. Cumulative, unprotected exposure to UVA and UVB rays. This refers to those received while participating in frequent sporting activities, during peak sun intensity, or working out-doors many hours a day, or even frequent long walks around noon without sun protection.

Figure 1.2, "Sunburns and Skin Cancer," presents a view of how severe DNA damage from UVB rays contributes to skin cancer. More details on this process can be found in Chapter X, where you will also see information about the effects of cumulative, long-term sun exposure. For now, we'll keep the focus on sunburns.

Sunburns and Skin Cancer (Figure 1.2)

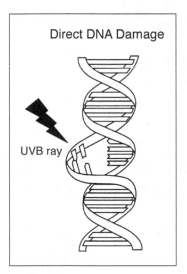

Direct DNA Damage

UVB ray

Overexposure to UV rays from the sun can result in sunburn, and sunburn can cause DNA damage. While our bodies do have a system of self-repair mechanisms to "clean up" the injury, sometimes it is simply unable to repair all of the "breaks" in the DNA or remove all of the damaged cells. As a result, these damaged skin cells eventually lose their ability to function normally. These cells—which behave abnormally—can lie dormant for years until they eventually manifest as skin cancer later in life. This is one reason why sunburns during childhood and teen years can contribute to certain forms of skin cancer in mid-life.

Overexposure: Sunburn Dangers

Now that we have learned that sunburns are the most important thing to avoid and that they can result in skin cancer years later, it is important to look at what actually happens when the skin is burned.

A severe burn over a large area of the body is dangerous and has ruined many vacations, even landing some people in the hospital. Sunburns can range from slight skin redness to blistering, painful burns. Depending on the severity of the burn, a mild to massive inflammation may result.

Sunburn, essentially, is the skin's reaction to excessive exposure to ultraviolet (UV) radiation, specifically UVB rays. Remember that UVB rays produce vitamin D, but these same rays can also burn the skin. Sunburn can sneak up on you, even on cold or cloudy days. It usually takes anywhere from a few hours to twenty-four hours for the skin to turn red or pink, which is the telltale sign of sunburn. Burned skin can be caused by a number of factors, including chemicals, fire, and excessive sun exposure.

Burned skin is classified in three degrees:

- First Degree: This involves the outer layer of skin (epidermis). In light-skinned people, the skin is red and may feel tender or painful. The skin will blanch white when touched. In dark-skinned people, redness may not be particularly noticeable, but the skin will feel tender.
- Second Degree: The skin has burned through to the second layer of skin (dermis) and will have a deep reddening, as well as swelling and blisters.
- Third Degree: The burn has penetrated the dermis and destroyed the nerve cells. This burn is typically not painful due to the destruction of nerve cells. A third-degree burn requires serious medical attention and can be especially dangerous if a large area of skin is involved. Third-degree burns caused by sun exposure are rare.

Besides the obvious skin tenderness and redness that result from a burn, headaches and fevers may also occur as the body works to fight the inflammation and often dehydration.

The risk of skin cancer is certainly one motivation for avoiding sunburns, and it is one of the key messages in this book. It is important to underscore another core message of this book: it is important for you and your family to be more mindful about the sun. Developing this mindfulness is like cultivating other daily habits such as brushing your teeth. It's that important! When you have a respectful relationship with the sun, you will be aware of its impact on your body. You will also be aware of the times when you can enjoy its warmth, and will notice when the sun's rays are too intense for your skin. By practicing sun sense, you and your family will be able to maximize the benefits of sun exposure without causing needless skin damage.

Respect the sun: don't get burned!

Key Points from Chapter 1 — The Sun: Friend or Foe?

- The sun is both a friend and a foe

- UVB rays burn the skin and produce vitamin D

- UVA rays promote tanning and do not burn the skin

- Both UVB and UVA rays can result in skin damage and increasing skin cancer risk

- Develop a Mindful relationship with the sun

- Moderate, safe sun exposure is healthy for most people, except in those who are especially sensitive to sun exposure

Chapter 2

Sun Sense

In the dead of winter, you wouldn't buy snow tires to drive around Miami. Nor would you pack scuba gear for a mountain hike in the Andes. When it comes to the sun, however, we too often listen to public health officials, bloggers, and doctors (both conventional and alternative) who offer broad-based advice that has nothing to do with our particular needs—advice such as:

"Don't go out in the sun between 10 a.m. and 4 p.m."

"Spend fifteen minutes in the sun a few times a week, and you'll make plenty of vitamin D"

"If you're outdoors during the summer, you'll make enough vitamin D for the winter"

The first bit of advice—about staying out of the hot, midday sun—is presented by public health experts whose aim is to protect the greatest number of people in the general population from sunburns. The second recommendation, to spend fifteen minutes in the sun to create vitamin D, is useless if you apply it in a time and place where it is impossible to obtain vitamin D–producing UVB rays. And the third statement, about tapping the summer sun for your vitamin D needs in the winter, is so indefinite that it does not apply to a significant number of people, especially those who live in far northern latitudes. What's more, none of these statements helps you make decisions based on your individual situation.

To make those personal decisions—and to know when to avoid the sun's damage and when to tap into its benefits—it is essential to develop sun sense. Just as you automatically know what to do when it rains—grab an umbrella, slow down while driving, stay away from lightning —so too must you develop safe sun practices in your local environment. This goes beyond just slapping on sunscreen when you're outdoors. Instead, what I am suggesting is to make a connection with the sun and learn how it impacts your body. Foster an awareness of the sun from the moment you step out into the daylight. That's real sun sense.

It would be convenient if I had a one-size-fits-all answer for my patients and others when they ask, "How much sun is safe?" Unfortunately, no such single answer exists. To truly answer that question, it is especially important to know and understand these top three factors:

- the basics of how sunlight works
- your position on the planet
- your individual skin type

Other factors, such as age, diet, medications, and genetic predisposition can also affect the amount of sun exposure that may be safe. But this chapter will focus on explaining how sunlight works and how to define your place on the planet relative to the sun; that, in itself, is a multilayered issue that considers not only the latitude and altitude where you are located but also the season of the year, the time of day, and weather conditions. The next chapter will explain the importance of knowing your skin type when making individual decisions about sun exposure.

To help build confidence in your own level of sun sense, this next section presents the fundamental facts about the nature of sunlight and how it reaches you across vast stretches of space.

Sun Sense: Know Your Locale

The more you know about the environment in your local area, the more confident you will feel about exposing your skin to the sun when it's appropriate. Where I live, in the San Francisco Bay area, heavy fog can block the sun's rays for significant amounts of time in the summer. But if you were to drive just 10 miles east of San Francisco, you could find yourself in bright sunshine—even when the city is socked in with fog. This means that people who live in sunnier areas have more opportunities to bask in vitamin D–producing UVB rays than those of us in the fog belt. In both areas, however, it is important to protect the skin from unnecessary UV exposure. That is why I stress that you must pay attention to conditions in your particular location, whether you are at home or on vacation, and not rely on generalized advice about sun exposure that may or may not apply to you.

Sun-Sense Essentials

Given that more than one million Earths could fit inside the sun, it seems a little naive to think that we can completely understand how the solar center of our universe really works. What we can do, however, is to grasp the essentials about how the sun interacts with our planet. And just as you may have learned about calorie calculations to make smarter diet decisions, you can also familiarize yourself with a few scientific concepts in order to better connect with the sun.

To make these concepts a little easier to remember, I have created the acronym "UP-LAST." Each letter in this acronym represents an environmental factor to consider when stepping outside during daylight hours. Understanding how sunlight works will give you a strong foundation for making decisions about whether or not—or when and where—to expose your skin to the sun. In the section below, we'll further examine what those letters stand for.

The six UP-LAST keys to developing sun sense:

1. ultraviolet rays
2. pollution and cloud cover
3. latitude
4. altitude
5. season of the year
6. time of day

Let's examine each of these UP-LAST factors individually:

1. Ultraviolet Rays—UVAs and UVBs

As noted in Chapter 1, the UVB rays emanating from the sun activate vitamin D production in the skin; but excessive exposure to these particular rays may also cause serious skin-damaging sunburns that can lead to skin cancer.

The other ultraviolet rays that are important to know about are UVA rays, which are responsible for tanning the skin, and like UVB rays, excessive exposure results in skin damage that may lead to future skin cancer.

But what exactly are UVB and UVA rays?

The sun emits rays that are part of the electromagnetic spectrum, a name given to the range of all possible frequencies and corresponding wavelengths of electromagnetic radiation. Among the shorter wavelengths on that spectrum are X-rays and gamma rays. On the other side of the spectrum, you will find the longer wavelengths, including radio waves (yes, the same ones broadcasters use for radio shows) and microwaves, which we've harnessed to quick-cook food. (See Figure 2.1 "Electromagnetic Spectrum.")

Electromagnetic Spectrum (Figure 2.1)

Electromagnetic Spectrum

Short wavelengths			UVC 100-280 nm	UVB 280-315 nm	UVA 315-400 nm		Long wavelengths	
Cosmic	Gamma Rays	X-Rays	Ultraviolet (UV) non-visible			Visible	Infrared	Microwave

credit: Kathy Rehak

Somewhat shorter than microwaves are the wavelengths that produce light visible to the human eye. Visible light allows us to see what is physically before our eyes in the form of shapes and objects, and it is composed of the seven cardinal colors of the rainbow: red, orange, yellow, green, blue, indigo, and violet.

The part of the spectrum known as ultraviolet, which is usually abbreviated as "UV," has a wavelength even shorter than that of visible light. These invisible UV rays are at the center of action when it comes to the sun's impact on our bodies. UV rays are further subdivided into three wavelengths, which are referred to as UVA, UVB, and UVC, or ultraviolet C, which has the shortest wavelength of the three.

Note on Nanometers

The length of a UV ray is measured in nanometers, or "nm"; and one billion nanometers is equal to one meter.

The shortest of the UV rays—UVC rays—are the most potent and dangerous. Their wavelength runs from 100 to 280 nm. Scientists speculate that if UVC rays were to reach the earth, they would burn things to a crisp. Fortunately, these UVC rays are blocked by the earth's ozone layer—even though that layer has been depleted in some areas. (See the box on "Ozone and Ultraviolet Rays" for further details.)

However, scientists have harnessed UVC radiation for its germi-cidal capabilities and it is used in modern sanitation technologies to inactivate viruses, bacteria, and other microorganisms.

Next to the UVC rays are the UVB rays, with wavelengths ranging from 280 to 315 nm. The ozone layer blocks a significant amount of UVB rays, but some penetrate through the atmosphere, and in areas where the ozone layer is diminished, UVB rays are particularly intense, necessitating caution and extra skin protection.

The last of this group are UVA rays, which have the longest wave-lengths, ranging from 315 to 400 nm. The ozone layer does not effec-tively block UVA rays, and these rays impact our skin year-round no matter where we are or where we live. In fact, UVA rays constitute 95 percent of all ultraviolet radiation that hits the earth or our skin.

In terms of managing our UV exposure to maximize the benefits of the sun while minimizing its harm, we will focus on UVA and UVB rays throughout the discussions in this book. To help you dis-tinguish between these two types of rays, the following chart lays out a few things to keep in mind about each type.

UVB	UVA
• Produces vitamin D by interacting with the skin	• Does not produce vitamin D
• Stimulates melanin production, starting the tanning process	• Primarily responsible for tanning the skin by oxidizing melanin
• Mid-range wavelength	• Long wavelength
• Penetrates the top layer of skin (epidermis)	• Penetrates deep into second skin layer of skin (dermis)
• Can result in sunburn. (Think of the B in UVB as representing "burning.")	• Does not burn the skin. (Think of the A in UVA as representing "aging.")

UVB	UVA
• Causes cumulative damage	• Causes cumulative damage
• Causes fine facial lines	• Causes deep facial wrinkles
• Linked with skin cancers, both non-melanoma and melanoma	• Linked with skin cancers, both non-melanoma and melanoma
• Can cause eye damage such as cataracts due to excessive sun exposure	• Can cause eye damage, but not as severe as that of UVB rays
• 93 percent blocked by a sun protection factor (SPF) of 15	• Blocked effectively by very few sunscreen chemicals
• Is able to be blocked by chemical or mineral sun products	• More effectively blocked by minerals such as zinc and titanium
• Has little success in penetrating glass	• Has 50 percent success rate in penetrating glass
• Will not result in vitamin D production when a person is sitting in the sun in front of a window	• Blocked by car windshields treated for UVA rays (Note: most side car windows are not treated.)
• Blocked, mostly, if not all, by clouds and fog but can come through light cloud cover	• Only partially blocked by dense fog or cloud cover

Measuring Ultraviolet Rays: UV Index and UV Meters

How are you supposed to know what level of UV rays are present on a particular day? The following tools can be used to assess this invisible form of radiation and can help inform your decisions about sun exposure. The best way to access the UV Index in your area is through weather channels on your computer or cell phone for up-to-date readings. You can also purchase a handheld monitor for a quick assessment of the UV Index, though they are not as accurate as what you can get from online sources.

UV Index (UVI): The World Health Organization has devised the Ultraviolet Index (UVI) to predict the strength of UV rays in a particular geographic region. (See chart, Chapter 11.) The index assigns a numerical value to various sun-exposure categories, ranging from less than 2 to signify "low" concerns about UV radiation, to 11+, which represents an "extreme" warning about being outdoors. At 11+, no one should be spending extended periods of time in the sun. For those people with sensitive skin, even a few minutes of exposure at this level can burn the skin. The index reading for your area is likely to appear in the weather section of a local newspaper or in television and radio reports. You can also access this information by going to the Environmental Protection Agency's (EPA) website (https://www.epa.gov/sunsafety). You can enter your zip code to find out the UVI in your specific location. It will give you only the index for solar noon—that time during the day when the sun is directly overhead. The website of the National Weather Service also provides an overview of UV levels.

Ultraviolet (UV) Meters: A UV meter is a small, handheld device that usually measures only UVB rays. While some meters give readings for both UVAs and UVBs, for practical purposes, you only need the UVB measurement. Knowing the intensity of the UVB rays can help you in two ways:

1. If the rays are too intense, they can burn the skin. Knowing this will help you determine whether it is advisable or not to expose your particular skin type. It will also help you gauge the amount of time that you can expose your skin before risking sunburn.
2. If the UVB rays are not strong enough, no vitamin D will be produced. This will enable you to know when to expose your skin for vitamin D production. A UVB strength of 3 is the

minimum for producing an appreciable amount of vitamin D, and a strength of 4 to 6 is ideal for most skin types. At lower levels, the strength is safer, but it will also take a lot longer to produce vitamin D. Read more on this issue in Chapter 3, page 4.

This device is useful for monitoring both everyday sun exposure and more infrequent sunbathing. If I am outside and my meter indicates that the rays are strong enough in the spring or fall, I will roll up my sleeves and pant legs, when possible, to produce vitamin D. Otherwise, I don't bother with exposing my skin. And for those warm days when I can sunbathe, I not only check the intensity of UVB rays but I also monitor my exposure with a timer that will wake me if I lose track of time or fall asleep.

More Information on UV Monitors

Many UV monitors on the market are advertised as "ultraviolet light monitors," or, simply, "UVB monitors." Not only can you buy stand-alone monitors, but these devices are also finding their way into swimmers' watches and other sporting gadgets. I have personally tested dozens of products from different companies and have found that some are more accurate than others. That said, they're accurate enough to help you determine, on the spot, whether or not the UVB rays in your area are enough or too much to expose your skin.

Now that you have a basic understanding about the various types of ultraviolet rays—which is the first among six factors that can affect the amount of sunlight available to you—it's time to look more closely at the rest of the list. As mentioned in the earlier section, these environmental factors include ultraviolet rays, pollution and cloud covers, latitude, altitude, season of the year; and time of day (spelling out the acronym UP-LAST).

2. Pollution and Cloud Cover

While the UV Index can help us determine how much ultraviolet radiation the sun sends to Earth on a particular day, it may not account for atmospheric conditions such as pollution and cloud cover. But in developing your sun sense, it is important to pay attention to these external conditions. If you are interested in producing vitamin D from the sun, keep this in mind: pollution can significantly reduce the penetration of UVB rays. However, UVB rays can penetrate light cloud or fog cover, producing unexpected sunburns for some people. In addition, fog and pollution will not effectively block out UVA rays.

Remember: Your skin can burn on a cloudy day!

The serious impact of pollution on reducing the availability of vitamin D–producing UVB rays cannot be understated. In fact, the disfiguring disease rickets, in which bones do not develop properly because of vitamin D deficiency, first became noticeable during the Industrial Revolution when soot and dense black smog from factories prevented city children from getting enough sunlight. Currently, rickets is a problem throughout the world, especially in industrialized countries, and researchers point to air pollution as one of the reasons.

Since air pollution can block UVB rays, it might seem that clouds would do the same—but that is not always the case. On a clear, sunny day, the presence of fluffy, white cumulus clouds can actually reflect these rays, intensifying the dose of UV radiation to your skin. Also keep in mind that on dense, cloudy days, UVB rays are blocked but UVA rays cut through, causing unnecessary skin damage if your skin is exposed. For these reasons, I also protect my skin on foggy or cloudy days by wearing a hat, which is something I do just about every day. Once, I measured both UVA and UVB rays with a meter on a very foggy day at noon. The UVA rays registered at a significant strength while the UVB rays were blocked completely. So, whether you are seeking the sun for vitamin D or staying out of it to avoid sunburns, pay attention to pollution levels and don't let the presence of clouds lull you into a false sense of security.

If You Squint, That's a Hint!

If the cloud cover is not thick, UVB rays can get through. If you squint, that's a hint! It means that UV radiation is coming through and may result in sunburn if your skin is unprotected.

3. Latitude

Unless you are an avid sailor, you have probably not given much thought to the concepts of latitude and longitude since learning about them in grammar school. When it comes to monitoring radiation from the sun, however, latitude is an important consideration.

If you look at a map (Figures 2.2 and 2.3), the latitude lines are the ones that run horizontally across the page as they show measurements for the angular distance from Earth's equator, which is marked as zero degrees (0°) latitude. The South Pole is 90°S (south) and the North Pole is 90°N (north). Longitude lines are the vertical lines on a map (they are omitted in the illustrations in this chapter).

The latitude for the San Francisco area where I live is 37° N—meaning it is 37 degrees north of the equator—and New York City can be found at 40° N. The southernmost tip of the United States is Key West, Florida, at latitude 24° N, and one of the northernmost cities in the country, Anchorage, Alaska, is at latitude 61° N.

The following chart will give you a sense of various latitudes around the world.

Latitudes of Major Cities in the World

City	Latitude	City	Latitude
St. Petersburg, Russia	59° N	New Delhi, India	28° N
Moscow, Russia	55° N	Hong Kong, China	22° N
Berlin, Germany	52° N	Mexico City, Mexico	19° N
London, England	51° N	Manila, Philippines	14° N
Vancouver, Canada	49° N	Bangkok, Thailand	13° N
Paris, France	48° N	EQUATOR	0°
Barcelona, Spain	41° N	Jakarta, Indonesia	6° S
Istanbul, Turkey	41° N	Lima, Peru	12° S
Beijing, China	39° N	São Paulo, Brazil	23° S
Athens, Greece	37° N	Johannesburg, South Africa	26° S
Tokyo, Japan	35° N		
Cairo, Egypt	30° N	Buenos Aires, Argentina	34° S
		Sydney, Australia	34° S

Latitudes of Major U.S. Cities

City	Latitude	City	Latitude
Seattle, WA	47° N	Charlotte, NC	35° N
Portland, OR	45° N	Los Angeles, CA	34° N
Boston, MA	42° N	Dallas, TX	32° N
Detroit, MI	42° N	San Diego, CA	32° N
Chicago, IL	41° N	Savannah, GA	32° N
New York, NY	40° N	Houston, TX	29° N
Denver, CO	39° N	New Orleans, LA	29° N
Washington, DC	38° N	Miami, FL	25° N
San Francisco, CA	37° N		

Use the maps in this section to check the latitude where you live. (See Figure 2.2, "Latitude Lines in the United States," and Figure 2.3, "Global Latitude Lines.") The world map may come in handy for those people lucky enough to travel to tropical regions. If you live in the United States, you will be able to determine your latitude within a couple of degrees.

Latitude Lines in the United States (Figure 2.2)

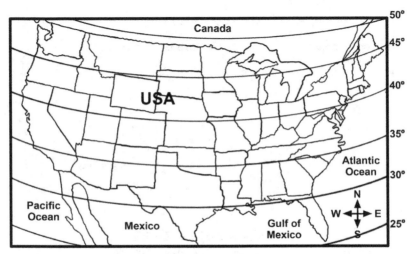

Global Latitude Lines (Figure 2.3)

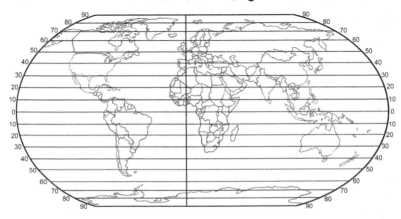

Besides using these maps or consulting an atlas, you can also find your exact latitude location by visiting the following website where you can plug in your zip code to get that information: https://getlatlong.net/. The first number that pops up is the latitude, and the second number is longitude, but for the purpose of evaluating sun-exposure issues, the latitude is the relevant number.

The Connection Between Vitamin D and Your Latitude

To understand the significance of these latitude numbers on the maps above, keep in mind that vitamin D–producing UVB rays are strongest at midday. So those walks in the early morning or late afternoon at higher latitudes will not produce vitamin D.

However, depending on where you are on the planet and the season of the year, the sun may not ever be directly overhead. At the

NOTE: UVB rays are at their peak when they are directly overhead.

equator, the latitude is 0°, and the sun is close to overhead all year long, which is why it is hot and humid in the tropics and the UVB strength at solar noon is intense year-round.

The term "vitamin D winter" was coined to illustrate that for those who live in northern latitudes, no vitamin D production will occur during certain months—generally October through March—although in some parts of world, this "winter" lasts even longer. This fact underscores why you should not assume that your blood level of vitamin D is optimal, let alone adequate, if you simply follow the very general advice to "spend fifteen minutes a day in the sun" to build vitamin D stores.

Again, see Figure 2.2 or 2.3 to find the latitude for your general area. You will refer to this information later—first, in the section below that discusses seasons of the year, and later, in Chapter 4, when you begin to determine your own parameters for safe sunbathing.

Zones of Latitude

Below are zones of the world divided into four categories by latitude:

0 to 23° = tropics
23 to 35° = subtropics
35 to 50° = mid-latitudes
50 to 70° = high latitudes

As you can see, each zone has a wide range of latitude difference. Knowing your zone will not necessarily help you make decisions regarding sun exposure. For instance, at latitude 23° you will be exposed to much more vitamin D–producing rays (UVBs) than latitude 34°, both of which are in the subtropical zones. Other tools that we will explore later in this book while discussing sensible sun exposure will help you make decisions about being outdoors, given specific latitudes.

4. Altitude

Latitude is one reference point for determining your distance from the sun; altitude is another. The sun's UV rays do not have to travel through as much of the atmosphere to reach Earth's high elevations, as they do to reach areas located below sea level. Consequently, if you live, ski, or hike in mountainous regions, you must be extra vigilant about sun exposure because UV rays are more intense at higher altitudes.

Snow poses another risk to be aware of in the mountains, since ultraviolet radiation intensifies when the sun's rays reflect off of snow. The EPA estimates that, in terms of overall UV radiation, fresh white snow reflects as much as 80 percent of the sun's rays, while sand reflects only 15 percent, and water reflects 10 percent.

Besides protecting your skin when UV rays reflect off of ground surfaces, it is also important to protect your eyes. (See Chapter 11 for guidelines on eye protection.)

5. Season of the Year

Just as you must figure out your latitude and altitude in calculating how much sun exposure is beneficial, consider the season of the year as well. We do not get the same amount of UVB rays year-round. As the seasons change, so does the angle of the sun's rays. Earth is tilted on its axis as it orbits annually around the sun. Summer occurs in the north when the Northern Hemisphere is tilted toward the sun, during which time the Southern Hemisphere experiences winter, and vice versa. In winter, the sun is lower in the sky at an increased angle. The angle causes more UVB rays to be blocked by the ozone layer. This process is illustrated in Figure 2.4, "The Seasons and the Sun."

As mentioned previously, during the winter, virtually no UVB rays penetrate the atmosphere in the more northern latitudes. If you live above 32°N latitude (for example, San Francisco or New York City, as well as St. Louis, Missouri, or Nashville, Tennessee), you will not be able to produce vitamin D during the winter months (or roughly from October to March). However, New Yorkers going to Florida for winter vacations or Seattle residents who travel to Mexico can be exposed to UVB rays that will give them a dose of vitamin D—or a sunburn—depending on how they manage their exposure.

Further, while many people believe that being out in the summer sun will give them an adequate supply of vitamin D for the winter, that is not necessarily the case. A number of studies have shown that the supply of vitamin D produced by summer sunbathing can fade even before the winter sets in. (Chapter 4 provides more details on producing vitamin D from the sun and other sources.)

When it comes to recognizing seasonal changes, your wardrobe no doubt reflects your awareness of these yearly cycles in Earth's calendar. By increasing your sun sense about the seasons, you will only deepen that awareness and become more empowered in your health decisions.

The Seasons and the Sun (Figure 2.4)

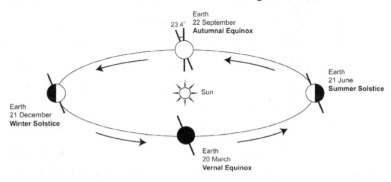

6. Time of Day

The angle (or degree) at which the sun's rays travel on their way to Earth not only changes across different seasons but it also varies during the day. In the early morning or late afternoon, when shadows are long, the sun's rays come in at a different angle than at solar noon, when the sun is directly overhead. At solar noon, the sun is at 90 degrees. If it is before or after solar noon, the angle decreases. The greater the angle, the more atmosphere the UV light must travel through. Remember, UVB rays diminish when they have farther to travel. In early morning or late afternoon, therefore, it is not possible to produce much, if any, vitamin D. This is especially true in higher latitudes.

Solar noon is the time of day when the sun is highest in the sky—even though it may or may not be noon according to the clock.

Also, solar noon can vary during the year because of changes in the speed of Earth's orbit around the sun. In the United States, daylight saving time also changes solar noon.

While considering the time of day, you should also remember that other factors impact the strength of UVB rays. For instance, clouds and air pollution can significantly reduce vitamin D production even when the sun is directly overhead. At the same time, in areas of clear sky, including the mountains or beach, more UVB rays will come through, creating more opportunities for building vitamin D. However, the sun is also more intense, and so extra precautions are needed to prevent sunburn. On extremely clear, cloudless days, or in places where sand and/or water increase reflection, it's important to eliminate or greatly minimize exposure in the hours around solar noon, when the UVB rays are at their strongest.

Practicing Sun Sense

In the process of writing this book, my own sun sense has deepened to a point where I am keenly mindful of the sun on a daily basis. It has also brought me back to feeling a deeper connection as a human being, enjoying and living with the sun just as my ancestors did—without fear but with awareness. Our ancestors got up with the sun and went to bed after sunset. Their lives revolved around the sun dictating planting and harvest seasons.

Sailors, traditionally, have used the sun to navigate through unknown waters; farmers, too, have always respected the sun's power—whether to nourish crops or cause them to wither. And, just as people throughout history have known how to read the sun and the stars, so can you.

Paying attention to the sun may be a new experience, and you might be surprised by your sudden awareness of how much the sun impacts you. As you progress through this book and begin to take more notice of your natural environment, you will deepen your connection with the sun. Once you've completed the next chapter about skin sense and put it together with what you've learned in this chapter, you will be well on your way to establishing your own personal approach to enjoying the sun.

Key Points from Chapter 2 — Sun Sense

- Your skin will only produce vitamin D under the right circumstances

- It is important to know your individual skin type

- Light skin produces vitamin D faster than dark skin

- UVB rays are strongest at midday

- Pollution and cloud cover decrease UVB rays

- Higher altitudes increase the strength of UVB rays

Chapter 3

Skin Sense

The skin is the largest organ in the body. In fact, it measures approximately 20 square feet, making it as large as a king-size bedspread and far larger than the heart, which is about the size of your fist. Your skin also sends a constant flow of information to other parts of the body, information that is vital to the functioning of the brain and other organs. Yet rarely do we regard the skin with the same level of esteem that we give to major organs such as the brain or the heart.

Certainly, when something goes wrong—such as a wrinkle, a pimple, or a cut—we apply herbal salves, expensive creams, or antibiotic ointments to the surface of our bodies. What we usually don't appreciate, however, is the complexity of the neural, hormonal, and immunological activities that go on within the skin.

To develop skin sense, then, it is important to recognize just how many vital roles the skin plays in your body. First and foremost, our skin protects us from the elements, both insulating us against the cold and cooling us with perspiration. It also forms a crucial barrier that blocks bacteria from entering our bodies.

In addition to its protective function, the skin's extensive network of nerve sensors is central to our sense of touch. On one end of the spectrum, our skin registers pain, which warns us away from many dangers. And the sensations of burning or itching instantly telegraph a "get away!" message to the brain. At the other end of that sensory spectrum, the skin also sends our body signals from soothing caresses, such as those that bond mothers to their babies. From this point, according to our customs and cultures, as we develop, we expect and crave various forms of pleasant stimulation on our skin, ranging from a handshake with a new acquaintance, to the hug that greets an old friend, to the sensual stroking by which we initiate lovemaking. It is through our skin that we perceive the sensations that fill our hearts with joy and sublime bliss.

In a far less romantic role, the skin also manufactures several hormones, including vitamin D, which, as noted in Chapter 1, actually *is* a type of hormone in its active form. Having the ability to create a hormone means that the skin is also capable of functioning as part of the endocrine system, similar to the thyroid or pituitary gland. Medical researchers are busy investigating these hormones that will lead to more discoveries about how this organ impacts the functioning of our bodies. Given all of its capabilities, we can begin to appreciate the special place that this organ we call skin occupies within our physiology.

In this chapter, you will first learn the basics of how your skin works before identifying your individual skin type and determining how it responds to the sun. This information will help you develop your skin sense, which can be combined with your sun sense so that you can make commonsense decisions about sun exposure. Remember that your ultimate goal is to be able to enjoy the warmth of the sun as well as its other benefits, such as vitamin D production, without damaging your skin and possibly triggering skin cancer.

The Skinny on Skin

To get some idea of how vast your skin's cellular network is, consider this: each square inch of your body has more than nine million skin cells. And those millions of cells are generally very busy—as cells from just below the outer layer of the skin constantly reproduce and push old cells up to the surface where they are sloughed off. Though sources vary, we shed approximately one billion skin cells each day, and the entire outer skin layer (epidermis) is replaced by new cell growth approximately every forty-eight days.

While it appears to be one smooth surface, your skin is actually composed of three major layers:

1. The epidermis: This top layer is a paper-thin, outside sheath.
2. The dermis: This more-sensitive layer lies just below and is protected by the epidermis.
3. The subcutis: This third and innermost layer is also called the subcutaneous fat layer, or hypodermis.

Let's take a closer look at each of these major skin layers.

Structure of the Skin (layers ans cells) (Figure 3.1)

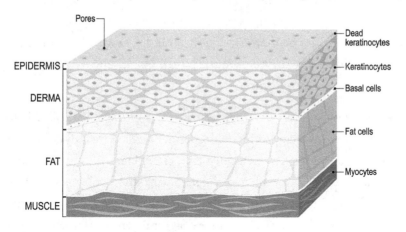

Epidermis

The epidermis is the outer skin layer. The epidermis retains water, yet it is waterproof and provides protection from environmental hazards. While the epidermis is about as thin as a pencil line in most parts of the body, it is nevertheless complex. This major skin layer is further subdivided into five layers and vitamin D is produced within these layers.

Another important fact about the epidermis is that it contains various types of cells, four of which are of particular interest in terms of the sun's impact on the body. These cells are squamous cells, basal cells, melanocytes (which contain melanin), and keratinocytes. Here are the main points to remember about the cells of the epidermis:

Basal Cells: These living cells line the bottom level (or base) of the epidermis (stratum basale), which is located just above the dermis. Basal cell carcinoma, the most common skin cancer, originates here.

Squamous Cells: These thin, flat cells originate from the lowest layer of the epidermis (the basal layer) and are found on the outer level (stratum corneum) of the epidermis, the part of the skin you see. As these cells migrate up toward the skin's surface, they mature and eventually die before they are sloughed off during the skin's monthly regeneration process. Squamous cells can give rise to squamous cell carcinoma, the second-most common form of skin cancer.

Melanocytes: Located along the bottom layer of the epidermis. Melanocytes are cells that produce skin pigment called melanin, and it is formed from tyrosine, an amino acid. People with light and dark skin have the same number of melanocytes. Skin color is based on what kinds of melanin and how much of each type the melanocytes produce. Two types of melanin exist—eumelanin and pheomelanin—and it is the ratio of these two pigments that give us the variety of colors that we see in skin tone:

  ▪ Eumelanin skin color is brown to black and protects against the sun's rays by limiting the amount of ultraviolet penetration (especially UVB rays) into the skin. Eumelanin further protects the body by "scavenging" the DNA-damaging free radicals (unstable atoms) that radiation produces in sun-exposed skin. Eumelanin is the most common melanin that allows people's skin to tan. Some people have dominant eumelanin, while others have dominant pheomelanin, such as those with very light skin and red hair, and will not tan at all. Methods to avoid skin burn and allow for safe tanning will be discussed in Chapter 11.

- Pheomelanin is yellow to red and is the form of melanin found in people who have red hair and light skin. Typically, women have more pheomelanin. This type of melanin cell produces a reddish tan, and for those people who have almost all pheomelanin cells, the skin burns very easily.

As mentioned earlier, the interaction between the sun's UVA rays and the skin stimulates melanocytes to produce a tan. The areas of our bodies that get the most sun exposure have the highest number of melanocytes—shoulders and upper back, followed by arms and lower back. The darker the skin (through tanning or genetics), the more its melanin protects it against sunburn. If repeated sunburns significantly damage the melanocytes, the risk of developing melanoma increases.

After age forty, our melanocytes decline in number and efficiency by 10 to 20 percent every decade, and the melanocytes that remain become less efficient in tan production. Consequently, our risk of sunburn goes up as we age, so it is increasingly important to develop new habits that protect us from overexposure.

Keratinocytes: Keratinocytes are the most common type of skin cells, and they are primarily mature squamous cells with some basal cells. They are found in the outermost layer of the epidermis. They make keratin, a protein that provides strength to skin, hair, and nails. For this reason, non-melanoma skin cancers such as basal cell carcinoma and squamous cell carcinoma are sometimes called keratinocyte cancers. The most common type of keratinocyte cancer is basal cell carcinoma. Keratinocytes form in the deep, basal cell layer of the skin and gradually migrate upward, becoming squamous cells before reaching the surface of the skin over the course of a month.

NOTE: There are two categories of skin cancer: melanoma and non-melanoma. Basal and squamous cell carcinomas are non-melanoma skin cancers. All types of skin cancers can develop anywhere on the body, especially sun-exposed areas. If basal and squamous cell carcinomas are detected early, these forms of cancer are treated easily, with the cure rates approaching 95 percent. However, if these cancers develop on the eyelid, nose, or mouth, the treatment can be quite extensive, which underscores the importance of regularly protecting your face and head from ultraviolet radiation. Melanoma, the most serious form of skin cancer, also has a high cure rate when caught and treated early, but surgeries to remove melanomas are more extensive.

Dermis

The dermis is the middle layer of skin, and it is much thicker than the epidermis. It contains collagen and elastin, which adds firmness and elasticity to the skin, giving the taut, firm appearance of youth. This layer also contains blood vessels, nerve fibers, glands, chemical messengers, hormones, and hair follicles.

Subcutaneous (subcutis)

The subcutaneous is the fat layer, or hypodermis. It is the third and deepest layer, forming a network of collagen and fat cells that fills out the skin, giving it a youthful appearance. It also provides insulation to retain body heat and cushions the body's organs from injury.

Now that you've learned a little about how the body's outer covering works for humans in general, it is time to move into the next section, which will describe what the sun can do to the skin based on your own individual body.

NOTE: In later decades of life, we lose the skin collagen in the dermis and subcutaneous layers and the skin can appear wrinkled and less firm. In areas of the body that have been subjected to years of sun exposure without protection, these areas show the most damage. Both UVB and UVA rays damage collagen. People with naturally dark skin suffer less skin damage than their Caucasian counterparts.

Skin Types and Tans

No one, among the billions of people on the planet, has your precise DNA. Not even identical twins have identical DNA. However, you do share many characteristics with others in the human gene pool who spring from common ancestors. Your eyes or hair, for instance, may reflect the colors that are predominant in your ethnic group.

When it comes to the skin, your heritage can affect how—or if— your skin tans or burns. To truly develop skin sense, then, it is crucial to know what your skin type is, as defined by both your genetic makeup and your body's reaction to the sun.

These skin types are not like the arbitrary color shades found at a makeup counter or in the paint department of a home improvement store. Rather, the skin typing charts commonly used throughout the medical profession and by government policy makers are based on research by Thomas B. Fitzpatrick, a Harvard Medical School doctor who conducted sun exposure tests in the early 1970s.

The scale developed from Fitzpatrick's work is known as the Fitzpatrick Classification Scale, and it identifies six different skin types based primarily on a person's genetic characteristics and the way his or her skin responds to the sun. By knowing your skin type, you will be better able to gauge how much sun exposure you can tolerate before being sunburned. Skin color can range from very white to very dark blue-black. In the United States, we have a melting pot of mixed heritages. For instance, I am Portuguese (a typically dark skin), French, Irish, and Scottish (generally light skin). My skin will burn easily if I do not have a tan first, but I can develop a dark, deep tan. My skin type is type 3. I keep my skin at a light tan to minimize unnecessary skin damage since my main interest in sun exposure is for vitamin D production.

Remember: NEVER allow your skin to burn

Fitzpatrick's six basic skin types and their basic tendencies include:

Type 1: Always burns, never tans, may freckle

Type 2: Burns easily, barely tans

Type 3: Sometimes burns, gradually tans

Type 4: Burns minimally, always tans

Type 5: Rarely burns, tans profusely

Type 6: Never burns, deeply tans

So which skin type are you? Knowing your skin type will obviously be important when making decisions about whether it's safe for you to be out in the sun—particularly if you choose to do what I call "sensible sunbathing," a concept you'll learn more about in Chapter 4. In addition, commercial sunscreen manufacturers consider skin types in designing their products, and the Food and Drug Administration (FDA) uses them as guidelines for a variety of policies, such as regulations for indoor tanning facilities. If you are not quite sure about your skin type, you can do a self-assessment test at the end of this chapter, which is adapted from the questionnaire developed by the Skin Cancer Foundation.

While skin type gives you a general picture of how your body responds to the sun, you can refine that information further by knowing about your individual MED—that is, your minimal erythemal dose—a concept that is explained in the next section.

Don't Turn Red; Know Your MED

Just as a good cook knows when to turn the oven off to avoid spoiling dinner, so too must you know how long you can expose your skin without getting burned. Understanding the scientific term *minimal erythemal dose*, or MED, as it pertains to sunburned skin, is one tool that may help you make that determination.

The word *erythema* comes from the Greeks and means "flush." It refers to the reddening of the skin caused by an increased blood flow to the microscopic blood vessels near the surface of the skin. Erythema can occur for multiple reasons, including sunburn, infections, and even standing too close to a campfire.

Basically, anything that increases heat to the skin can result in erythema.

One minimal erythemal dose (or 1-MED) is the term researchers and doctors use to describe the minimum amount of UVB that produces skin redness or pink within twenty-four hours after exposure. This standardized measurement helps the medical profession determine appropriate levels of UVB treatment for conditions such as psoriasis. Typically, a doctor might expose a small area of a patient's skin to UVB light to determine 1-MED for that person (since a lighter-skinned patient will need to start treatments at a weaker dose than a darker-skinned individual). Both the indoor tanning industry and sunlamp manufacturers also refer to standard MED measurements in their services and products. Heat from the sun (or a UVB light source) can sometimes produce immediate, temporary skin redness. Therefore, doctors will wait twenty-four hours to check the skin to determine if the reaction is due to the dose of UVB exposure when it is used as part of a treatment protocol.

Minimal Erythemal Dose (MED): The threshold dose of UVB exposure that it takes to produce a redness on the skin within twenty-four hours after exposure.

Research by Michael Holick showed that exposure of 85 percent of the body to one minimal erythemal dose of UV radiation (slight pinkness to the skin after twenty-four hours of exposure) may produce 10,000 to 25,000 IU. It is likely rare to produce over 10,000 IU of vitamin D in one day unless you are a young person. The older we are the less vitamin D will be produced by the skin.

So, if your skin burns three hours after exposure, you have gone way beyond your MED. To be safe, you should not expose your skin any longer than half of your MED. Interestingly, according to researcher Michael Holick, the skin is not capable of producing vitamin D once it has reached its MED.

Okay, so how are you supposed to know what your MED is? Unfortunately, no hard-and-fast rules exist to help you determine your MED because skin types vary by individual. And because your MED changes depending on the intensity of the sun, you will need to be aware of other factors—such as the latitude and intensity of UVB rays at different times of the year—to determine how long to expose your skin. Therefore, it is very important for you to know your body, pay attention to its signals, and recognize how it reacts to the sun.

No matter what you do, exposing your skin is not an exact science. And when in doubt, get out of the sun. This is simply a framework for how to think about sun exposure. Having an idea of your MED is simply a tool among many others that are offered in this book. Here's one guideline to keep in mind: If you ever feel that sense of "burning" on your skin when you're outdoors, trust it. Cover up or go inside. The burning sensation is different from the feeling of warmth from the sun that everyone enjoys. However, we don't always know when our skin is burning, and sunburn may not show up for twenty-four hours. This is where common sense comes in. When in doubt, protect until you feel confident that you know your personal MED.

If your skin *ever* turns pink or red after sun exposure, skin damage occurred! You were out too long!

Example: In my particular situation, I live at the thirty-seventh latitude in the San Francisco Bay area. I know that in the middle of summer on a clear day with a UV Index of 5 or 6, I can safely expose my skin for fifteen minutes without my skin turning pink twenty-four hours later. On the other hand, if I travel to a mountainous area at a higher altitude or travel to a tropical region at a lower latitude, I will have to adjust my time in the sun since the UVB rays will be much more intense in those places.

In the sun-exposure section, I will lay out all of these tools so that you will have a good reference guide to skin protection and safe sun-exposure protocols.

Mind Your MED

Here's another tidbit to remember: when the skin reaches its MED, vitamin D production stops. In fact, a vitamin D metabolite begins to destroy excess vitamin D. This is why a person cannot overdose on vitamin D from sun exposure.

Conscious Care for Your Skin

Advertisements constantly bombard us with messages about products we should buy to care for our skin. But what you really need for keeping this precious organ healthy does not simply come from a bottle or a tube. As you have seen in this chapter, giving your body the best care comes from developing your own skin sense. Understanding how your skin works, identifying your skin type, and determining the optimal time for you, personally, to enjoy the sun will make you more confident and conscious about the skin you're in.

Your Skin Type: A Self-Assessment Test

A SPECIAL NOTE: This quiz below is reprinted with permission from the Skin Cancer Foundation. Please note that this quiz uses the term "fair" to describe light skin. My preference is to use the words "light skin" as I have throughout this book.

"Where Does Your Skin Fit In?" Quiz

The Fitzpatrick Classification Scale is a skin classification system first developed in 1975 by Thomas Fitzpatrick, MD, of Harvard Medical School. His skin classifications and its adaptation are familiar to dermatologists. To determine your Fitzpatrick skin type, our quiz measures two components (genetic disposition and reaction to sun exposure). Types range from the very fair (Type 1) to the very dark (Type 6).

So, grab a piece of paper, sharpen your pencil, and take the quiz below to discover what your type is. Then read our analyses for some type-tailored sun-safety advice.

Part I: Genetic Disposition (circle your answer)

Your eye color is:

      0 = light blue, light gray, or light green
      1 = blue, gray, or green
      2 = hazel or light brown
      3 = dark brown
      4 = brownish black

Your natural hair color is:

      0 = red or light blonde
      1 = blonde
      2 = dark blonde or light brown
      3 = dark brown
      4 = black

Your natural skin color (before sun exposure) is:

        0 = ivory white
        1 = light or pale
        2 = light to beige, with golden undertone
        3 = olive or light brown
        4 = dark brown or black

How many freckles do you have on unexposed areas of your skin?

        0 = many
        1 = Several
        2 = A few
        3 = Very few
        4 = None

Total score for genetic disposition: _____

Part II: Reaction to EXTENDED Sun Exposure
    (circle your answer)

How does your skin respond to the sun?

        0 = always burns, blisters, and peels
        1 = often burns, blisters, and peels
        2 = burns moderately
        3 = burns rarely, if at all
        4 = never burns

Does your skin tan?

        0 = never
        1 = seldom
        2 = sometimes
        3 = often
        4 = always

How deeply do you tan?

       0 = not at all or very little
       1 = lightly
       2 = moderately
       3 = deeply
       4 = very deeply

How sensitive is your face to the sun?

       0 = very sensitive
       1 = sensitive
       2 = normal
       3 = resistant
       4 = very resistant/never had a problem

Total score for reaction to sun exposure: _____

**Add up your genetic disposition and sun exposure totals
to find your skin type: _____**

0 to 6 Points: **Type 1**—You always burn and never tan in
the sun. You are extremely susceptible to skin damage
as well as cancers such as basal cell carcinoma and
squamous cell carcinoma. You are also at very high risk
for melanoma, the deadliest type of skin cancer. Generally,
follow the Skin Cancer Foundation's prevention tips (check
www.skincancer.org) but use a sunscreen with an SPF of
30+ and clothing with a UPF rating of 30 or higher. Seek
the shade whenever you are out in the sun. Check your
skin head-to-toe each month, paying careful attention to
any suspicious growths, and make sure you have an annual
professional skin checkup.

7 to 12 Points: **Type 2**—You almost always burn and rarely tan in the sun. You are highly susceptible to skin damage as well as cancers such as basal cell carcinoma and squamous cell carcinoma. You are also at high risk for melanoma, the deadliest type of skin cancer. Generally, follow the Skin Cancer Foundation's prevention tips (check www.skincancer.org) but also consider using a sunscreen with an SPF of 30+ and clothing with a UPF rating of 30 or higher. Seek the shade whenever you are out in the sun. Check your skin head-to-toe each month, paying careful attention to any suspicious growths, and make sure you have an annual professional skin checkup.

13 to 18 Points: **Type 3**—You sometimes burn and sometimes tan in the sun. You are susceptible to skin damage as well as cancers such as basal cell carcinoma and squamous cell carcinoma. You are also at risk for melanoma, the deadliest type of skin cancer. Be sure to apply a sunscreen with an SPF of at least 15 every day, wear sun-protective clothing, and seek the shade between 10 a.m. and 4 p.m., when the sun is strongest. Check your skin head-to-toe each month, paying careful attention to any suspicious growths, and make sure you have an annual professional skin checkup.

19 to 24 Points: **Type 4**—You tend to tan easily and are less likely to burn. But you are still at risk; use sunscreen with an SPF of 15+ outside and seek the shade between 10 a.m. and 4 p.m. Follow all other Prevention Tips from the Skin Cancer Foundation as well. (See www.skincancer.org.) Check your skin head-to-toe each month, paying careful attention to any suspicious growths, and make sure you have an annual professional skin checkup.

25 to 30 Points: **Type 5**—You tan easily and rarely burn, but you are still at risk. Use sunscreen with an SPF of 15+ and seek the shade between 10 a.m. and 4 p.m. Acral lentiginous melanoma, a virulent form of the disease, is more common among darker-skinned people. These melanomas tend to appear on parts of the body not often exposed to the sun and often remain undetected until after the cancer has spread. Check your skin head-to-toe each month, paying careful attention to any suspicious growths, especially on the palms, soles of the feet, and mucous membranes. Make sure you have an annual professional skin checkup.

31+ Points: **Type 6**—Although you do not burn, dark-skinned people are still at risk for skin cancers and should wear sunscreen with an SPF of 15+ and seek the shade between 10 a.m. and 4 p.m. Acral lentiginous melanoma, a virulent form of the disease, is more common among darker-skinned people. These melanomas tend to appear on parts of the body not often exposed to the sun and often remain undetected until after the cancer has spread. Check your skin head-to-toe each month, paying careful attention to any suspicious growths, especially on the palms, soles of the feet, and mucous membranes. Make sure you have an annual professional skin checkup.

This skin-type quiz is for informational and entertainment purposes only. The content is not intended to be a substitute for professional medical advice, diagnosis, or treatment. Always seek the advice of your physician or other qualified health provider with any questions you may have regarding a medical condition.

Key Points from Chapter 3 — Skin Sense

- The skin is the largest organ in the body

- Excessive exposure to these particular rays may also cause serious skin-damaging sunburns, that can lead to skin cancer

- UVB rays produce vitamin D3 and can burn the skin

- UVA rays tan the skin

- UVB and UVA cause cumulative skin damage

- UVA rays are strongest in summer, but are also strong all year round

- UVB rays do not penetrate glass. UVA rays do penetrate glass

- Access the UV Index in your area is through weather channels

Getting Vitamin D from the Sun

Which of these two options provides the best vehicle for delivering vitamin C to your body: a fresh orange or a vitamin C supplement?

Answering that question can touch off any number of scientific debates, and your response to it will be affected by your individual health and life conditions. For most people, oranges are synonymous with vitamin C, or ascorbic acid. In addition, an orange also contains a complex of other nutrients that are rich in antioxidants, including bioflavonoids, pectin, vitamin A, hesperetin, naringin, and B-complex vitamins, as well as some calcium and potassium and the much-needed fiber.

Can Your Diet Help Prevent Skin Cancer?
(from SkinCancer.org)

"Studies have shown that substances called antioxidants, including vitamins and other nutrients, may help fight off free radicals and prevent the damage they do that can cause skin cancer. A 2002 study in the *Journal of Investigative Dermatology* found that UV exposure greases the wheels for skin damage partly by depleting antioxidants in the body. So, it makes sense that replacing these protective substances could bolster the weakened defenses."

By the same token, supplement pills can also deliver vitamin C to the body. They, too, can contain not only ascorbic acid but also some of the other constituents of the vitamin C complex. But pills can never exactly duplicate nutrients offered by an orange, which are important to our health. Clearly, even though oranges and vitamin pills can both supply vitamin C, personal circumstances and needs will shape decisions about which one is best for you to use.

When it comes to vitamin D, similar issues arise. Is it better for your dose of D to come from the sun? Should it come from food— or from a supplement? In reality, any of these sources can provide vitamin D. But I contend that, optimally, some of our supply of vitamin D should come from the sun. In fact, I would argue that, in some ways, getting vitamin D from the sun is similar to getting vitamin C complex from a whole food, such as an orange. Like the orange, which offers an array of health-giving vitamin C components, so, too, does the sun emit a range of matter that work together to maximize the production of vitamin D.

Recommending sensible sun exposure as a healthy choice is serious business and one that I do not make lightly or out of personal preference. However, after studying the science of vitamin D, as well as the issue of skin cancer, I believe it is both safe and healthy to tap the sun for some of our vitamin D—if and when it's possible— for sound reasons. Consider the following:

- Vitamin D production: Under the right conditions, one full-body dose (whole body exposed) of UVB rays from the sun can produce a significant dose of vitamin D. Some researchers claim that under the *right* conditions some people will produce as much as 10,000 to 25,000 IU of D3 in twenty to thirty minutes. While there are reports that some people could make 25,000 IU in one day, this would be a rare occurrence.

So, how much can be made in the proper conditions? That amount is probably closer to 10,000 IU, which is pretty amazing. Dr. Michael Holick is credited with these findings. Of note, the subjects involved were young adults with 85 percent of the body exposed to UVB rays.

- The assertion that we will produce enough vitamin D if we simply expose our arms and legs to sunshine for twenty minutes, three times a week is all that we need to produce a healthy amount of vitamin D. This belief is simply incorrect for most people, especially those furthest from the equator.

- Mother Nature's mysteries: While researchers have made enormous breakthroughs in understanding the benefits of vitamin D in the past couple of decades, we have barely scratched the surface in terms of knowing how the natural production of this vitamin ultimately impacts our bodies. As part of the natural production of D3, the sun's infrared rays also have known health benefits.

- Interestingly, in situations of extreme sun exposure, several studies have shown a protective benefit for the most virulent form of skin cancer, melanoma. Those who receive significant, chronic sun exposure, such as farmers or sailors, have less diagnoses of melanoma. However, these same people do have frequent diagnoses of basal cell carcinoma and squamous cell carcinoma.

In addition to D3, we are still learning about the hormones lumisterol and tachysterol that are produced from the sun's interaction with the skin. Arguably, just as scientists cannot replicate every attribute of breast milk in infant formula, a pill cannot fully reproduce all of the physiological reactions, hormones, or other substances that the sun creates when it interacts with the skin. Therefore, the sun's role in creating vitamin D in our bodies—and the undiscovered properties of sunlight itself—may aid us in ways that we simply have not yet recognized. In fact, early research on lumisterol stated it was basically not active after it assisted in the production of D3 in the skin. Now we understand that lumisterol can circulate in the blood and potentially accumulate in steroidogenic tissues such as the adrenal gland. This is another reminder that while we know a lot about the rays of the sun, we simply do not know everything.

Philosophically, my overall approach to health is that our food and other nutrients should come from the most unadulterated sources possible. Further, the most natural way human beings have evolved to produce vitamin D is through exposure to the sun and not from the intake of food—except perhaps for people living in extreme northern latitudes, such as Eskimos, whose traditional diets are high in fish oils laden with vitamin D.

In other words, it's better to get at least some of our D from sunshine—that is, from vitamin D–producing UVB rays. Having said that, however, I fully recognize that the vast majority of people in modern, technological societies or aged adults living indoors will not be able to receive the amount of vitamin D their bodies need if they rely on sunshine alone, nor will those who live in higher latitudes or who stay indoors when vitamin D–producing rays are available outdoors. The best option for most people is to responsibly expose their skin to the sun when UVB rays are present, test for vitamin D status, and supplement appropriately.

A Cautionary Note . . .

In their real concern to educate the public to take measures to prevent skin cancer, dermatologists, cancer organizations, and governmental agencies hammer us with the message that we should "shun the sun," and some even recommend that we obtain vitamin D only from food or supplements.

Unquestionably, protecting the skin is important, and I regularly see people looking like lobsters, despite all the warnings. Keep in mind that exposing the face is never recommended, and it should be protected, primarily with hats and secondarily with sunscreen. However, except in rare instances, most of us do not need to avoid the sun to such an extent that we miss the benefits of vitamin D and other hormones that prudent sun exposure can produce in our bodies. It is important to note that I use the word *prudent* to describe the type of sun exposure that is beneficial to your well-being.

Also, it is true that vitamin D–producing UVB rays can be obtained in some tanning salons and through the use of special lightbulbs. This chapter focuses on sun-produced vitamin D, and exposure to artificially produced UVB rays raises other concerns that are discussed in Chapter 11.

Along the path to making decisions regarding wise sun exposure for you and your family, your first step is to recognize the crucial role vitamin D plays in keeping you healthy. That is the focus of the next section.

Vitamin D—Get It Right

Vitamin D in its active form (calcitriol) has long been recognized as a substance that increases calcium and phosphorus absorption in the gut. And now, mounting research is showing that calcitriol can also help strengthen your immune system and lower the risks associated with multiple cancers, diabetes, Crohn's disease, and heart disease. In addition, vitamin D can help fight mental disorders as well as muscle and joint problems. The body, in fact, is loaded with receptors for vitamin D, from the brain, heart, and intestines to the thyroid, prostate, and mammary glands. Quite simply, vitamin D, in its active form, is critical for our bones and our overall health. It's that important. And because it is so important, it is crucial to get it right for our families and ourselves. That means we cannot be irresponsible about obtaining it. It is a mistake to think that spending a few haphazard minutes in the sun, drinking a glass of milk every day, or taking low-dose supplements will meet our body's demand for D. Nor should we regard D as a cure-all and start gobbling 10,000 IU daily as though it were the latest miracle pill fad. In Chapter 7, you will learn about vitamin D supplement recommendations.

The Myriad Benefits of Vitamin D

Active vitamin D (calcitriol) is one of the most important hormones for human health, and a deficiency of this powerful substance has been linked to numerous health issues including multiple forms of cancer, the common cold, diabetes, and even Parkinson's disease. There are vitamin D receptors (VDR) throughout the body and in all major glands. inAs noted in this chapter, and throughout the research community, one of the major biological functions of vitamin D is to promote the intestinal absorption of calcium and phosphorous. But vitamin D's benefits extend way beyond calcium and phosphorus absorption, and ongoing research continues to report more potential benefits.

Some of the known benefits of vitamin D:

- helps build and maintain healthy bone tissue
- acts as a natural anti-inflammatory
- functions as a powerful antioxidant, supporting cell maturation and health

- boosts immunity, helping stave off influenza and the common cold
- aids in the prevention of multiple forms of cancer
- supports brain development
- fosters mental health
- plays an essential role in fetal development in multiple ways
- stimulates the kidneys to reabsorb calcium
- builds strong bones, teeth, and nails
- supports the functioning of the nervous system
- promotes muscle and joint health
- supports thyroid and adrenal function
- helps maintain hearing acuity by promoting strength of inner ear bones
- supports maintenance of a balanced body weight
- functions as an essential component of visual acuity
- improves kidney function
- supports lung health and respiratory conditions
- supports heart health, including normal heartbeat
- helps maintain normal cholesterol levels
- supports maintenance of normal blood pressure
- assists in regulating blood sugar levels
- may prevent or reduce occurrence of Type 2 and possibly Type 1 diabetes
- supports healthy peripheral nervous system
- may be useful in the treatment of some cancers
- promotes skin development
- supports efficient blood clotting
- plays a role in balancing sex hormones in men and women
- functions as an essential component of fertility in both men and women

Vitamin D Builds Bones

One of the most critical roles of active vitamin D (calcitriol) is attributed to supporting bone health throughout our life, starting in the womb and lasting until our skeleton reaches peak bone mass around the age of thirty. After the age of thirty, vitamin D helps to maintain stable bone density. There are a host of nutrients that work together to build and maintain strong bones, but chief among them are vitamin D, calcium, and phosphorous. These rely on a healthy blood level of vitamin D to increase absorption of these nutrients.

Let's begin with a look at how the body develops healthy bones. During a woman's pregnancy, the forming fetal skeleton is composed of cartilage, which is much more flexible than bone. Cartilage begins developing into hard bone just prior to birth and continues hardening though adolescence and early adulthood. Healthy adult bone is hard yet slightly flexible.

A large part of bone formation and maintenance depends on calcium and phosphorus; if you do not have enough vitamin D, your bones cannot access these minerals. As an indication of just how vital vitamin D is to this process, remember this: in its active form as calcitriol, it increases calcium and phosphorous absorption by a whopping 50 percent in the intestines.

As a side note, in my research, I found that bones need a multitude of other nutrients to be healthy that are often ignored by many doctors, including vitamin C, vitamin K, potassium, magnesium, and vitamin B-12, just to name a few, as well as macronutrients in the right amount, such as proteins and healthy fats, which I expand upon in my book *Dr. Lani's No-Nonsense Bone Health Guide*.

Prolonged vitamin D deficiency can result in osteoporosis, rickets in children, and osteomalacia in adults, a condition that is

sometimes referred to as "adult rickets." These conditions are covered in Chapter 5 on deficiencies. Rickets, in fact, was the disease
that first helped researchers isolate and identify the substance we
now call vitamin D. To understand how scientific thinking about
vitamin D has evolved—and some of the medical controversies
about it that continue today—it is helpful to know a little history,
which I'll cover in the following section titled "A Brief History of
Vitamin D."

A Brief History of Vitamin D

During the late 1600s, in the newly developed urban centers
around Europe, parents began to see their small children dis-
figured by bowed or shortened legs and abnormally curved
spines. Some of these children were tortured by extreme muscle
cramps and bone pain; others failed to develop mentally. The
term *rickets* became associated with this condition at that time,
but the cause remained elusive. No one knew that these children suffered from a vitamin D deficiency.

It took more than two hundred years for scientists to make
the connection between these deformities and afflictions and
the upsurge in urban living, indoor factory work, and the thick,
light-occluding smog of the Industrial Revolution. Eventually,
however, in the early nineteenth century, Polish physician
Jędrzej Śniadecki observed that the children in rural areas
around Warsaw did not suffer from rickets. From that obser-
vation, he deduced that sunlight either cured or prevented the
condition—since the children in the countryside enjoyed ample
sunshine. In fact, sun exposure became one of the main treatments for rickets into the first few decades of the twentieth century. Photographs from that era show children basking in the

rays of the sun on hospital balconies, solariums, and even on boats, such as the Floating Hospital for Children that still exists in Boston today (although the hospital facility is no longer on a boat, but in buildings on shore). UVB lamps also came into vogue as a treatment for the disease during the first few decades of the twentieth century.

Around the same time as Śniadecki's discoveries, other researchers noted that cod liver oil (which is high in vitamins A and D) could also reverse rickets. The folklore of people living along the coasts of northern Europe also attested to the health benefits of cod liver oil; however, its use as an anti-rickets agent did not become widespread. A further discussion about cod liver oil can be found in Chapter 8).

Although rickets became treatable, it remained unchecked until the early part of the twentieth century. At that time, as industry boomed, and more people moved from farms to big cities in the United States and Europe, the incidence of rickets reached alarming proportions. By 1900, the disease was so common, it was estimated that an astonishing 90 percent of children in Leiden, the Netherlands, and 80 percent of children in Boston suffered from rickets. Then, in the 1920s, researchers confirmed that both sunshine and cod liver oil could treat rickets because of a single substance in both, a substance that was named "vitamin D"—even though researchers did not know at the time exactly what vitamin D was. It is worth noting that one of these researchers, Elmer McCollum, coined the term *vitamin D* when he separated and tested various elements found in cod liver oil.

A vitamin is defined as a substance that is essential for normal growth and nutrition and is required in the diet because a vitamin cannot be synthesized by the body. At the time of

McCollum's early experiments, the idea that the body could create vitamin D from sunlight had not become fully established; therefore, he called his discovery a vitamin. Today we know that there are more than fifty metabolites (forms) of vitamin D and, in its active form, it is a type of steroid hormone.

By 1924, public health officials launched a campaign to eradicate rickets by promoting sunlight therapy and the irradiation of foods. UVB rays were used to produce vitamin D in the food supply to boost everyone's level of vitamin D. From the 1930s through the 1950s, bread, milk, hot dogs, and even soft drinks and beer were among the various foods that were fortified with vitamin D, and rickets was virtually eliminated in the United States during the 1930s.

There was a defining moment regarding government-sanctioned recommendations for vitamin D during the 1950s. In that decade, it was thought that the over-fortification of milk with vitamin D was responsible for an outbreak of a condition called "hypercalcemia" in a group of infants. Hypercalcemia is when the blood level of calcium is dangerously elevated. This theory was ultimately never proven, but fears about this seeming "epidemic" led to a ban on fortifying foods with vitamin D in Europe at that time. Some researchers point to this event as the reason doctors continue to be leery of recommending higher doses of vitamin D today—a concern that is playing out in ongoing debates over the amount of vitamin D that should be included in the U.S. government's Recommended Dietary Allowance (RDA). Milk, it should be noted, is fortified in the United States, with the standard amount being 100 IU of vitamin D per 8-ounce glass—which may be enough to ward off rickets, but is only a fraction of dietary need. In fact, some researchers now argue that adults need a minimum of 4,000 to 5,000 IU of D daily from all sources, whether it is manufactured from sunshine or obtained through supplementation.

In the late 1960s and early 1970s, scientists began to understand that the substance labeled "vitamin D" was actually more akin to a hormone. They confirmed that biologically inactive vitamin D3 (cholecalciferol) eventually converts to its physiologically active form of vitamin D called calcitriol, or 1,25-D. Calcitriol is a potent type of steroid hormone. Yet, because the name "vitamin D" had been in use for so many years, it stuck.

Significantly, in the 1990s, researchers found that calcitriol is not only produced in the kidneys, it can also be formed within a variety of other cells in the body, including the breast, prostate, colon, brain, and skin. Dr. Michael Holick and his team of researchers at the Vitamin D, Skin, and Bone Research Laboratory at Boston University Medical Center were credited with this discovery, which had also been reported by European researchers. Some of the most exciting vitamin D research today centers on this autocrine signaling activity, which is defined as "a secretion of a cell that affects the cell itself" (according to the *Oxford Dictionary of Sports Science and Medicine*). In other words, vitamin D does not necessarily have to travel through the bloodstream to become useful to the body. The bulk of 25-D is released into the bloodstream from the liver it travels to the kidneys, where it converts to the biologically active form of vitamin D (1,25-D). Interestingly, some of the 25-D goes directly to other tissues in the body to transform into 1,25-D. This is known as autocrine function.

One other bit of history is worth noting about vitamin D. During the 1980s, stories about depletion of the UV-blocking ozone layer, and subsequent reports about the rise in skin cancer, led many people back indoors. This is one of the reasons vitamin D deficiencies are widespread today. And rickets, the centuries-old disease that originally spawned the search for vitamin D, is once again on the rise. Despite these developments, the conventional medical view today is that everyone should "shun the sun," and government reports label the sun as "carcinogenic." This view is beginning to change with new advice that ten minutes of sunshine on the arms and face three times a week is enough to produce ample vitamin D. You will see later in this book that this recommendation is woefully inadequate.

Certainly, no one should indulge in excessive exposure to UV radiation. And burning the skin should be absolutely avoided. But you must be clear about what you're missing when you completely avoid the sun: the powerful benefits of vitamin D and all of the other positive impacts the sun has on the body.

Vitamin D: Sunbeams in Your Bloodstream

At this point, you may recognize the value of producing some of your vitamin D via the sun. However, many names are used for vitamin D in all of its forms, and it can be very confusing. To make this terminology a little easier, refer to the chart below.

The following chart will help you keep track of the chemical names mentioned in the explanation of "How Your Skin Makes Vitamin D from the Sun." The chart also includes supplement forms of vitamin D. You'll often see those names in media, on supplement labels, or in online discussions about vitamin D.

Vitamin D Nomenclature

Name	Definitions
Pro-vitamin D 7-dehydrocholesterol Pro-hormone vitamin D	Vitamin D precursor. This form of cholesterol is found just under the top two layers of skin. When the skin is exposed to adequate UVB rays, those rays interact with 7-dehydrocholesterol and produce vitamin D3, or cholecalciferol.
Cholecalciferol Vitamin D3 (pre-hormone) Calciol Calciferol	Produced in the skin when the skin is exposed to ultraviolet (UVB) rays. Vitamin D3 activates the intestinal wall, increasing calcium and phosphorous absorption from the intestines into the bloodstream. On supplement labels, these are the names that can appear for vitamin D.
Prohormone Calcidiol 25-hydroxyvitamin D3 or 25-D3 25(OH)D3 Calcifediol 25-hydroxyergocalciferol or 25-D2 25-hydroxyvitamin D 25(OH)D	This form of vitamin D from sun exposure or oral ingestion travels to the liver where it is converted (hydroxylated) to 25-hydroxyvitamin D. The blood test to determine vitamin D status is the called 25-D test. On a lab request you may just see vitamin D or you might also see a breakdown of D2 and D3 This form of vitamin D is a pre-hormone that is produced in the liver by hydroxylation. 25-D2 originates from fungi that is exposed to UVB rays.
Calcitriol 1,25-dihydroxyvitamin D 1,25-D3 1,25-D2	1,25-D is the active form of vitamin D. It is a type of steroid hormone, technically a secosteroid hormone. It is produced in the kidneys from either 25-D2 or 25-D3. D3 (but not D2) is also produced through autocrine signaling, where it is produced elsewhere in the body, including the brain, thyroid, adrenal glands, and even in the skin itself.

Supplemental vitamin D3 Cholecalciferol* Calciferol	The primary sources for D3 supplements are from fish oil, lamb's wool, sheepskin, or the vegan source lichen.
	Fish oil is rich in D3, and it is extracted and made into supplements. Lanolin comes from lamb's wool or sheepskin. Cholesterol is extracted from the wool grease and wool wax alcohols obtained from the cleaning of wool after shearing. It is then irradiated with UVB rays to produce D3.
	A vegan source of D3 is produced by lichen that is a composite organism that arises from algae. This offers vegans a better source of vitamin D3 supplementation than ergocalciferol or D2.
	Cow's milk is typically fortified with vitamin D3 (100 IU per cup)
Ergocalciferol* Supplemental vitamin D2	Supplemental D2 is derived from yeast or fungi through irradiation with UVB rays. The human body does not produce D2.
	Non-dairy milk products are fortified with D2; thus it is considered the vegan form of vitamin D. D3 is two to three times more potent than D2.

Cholecalciferol is the best choice in supplemental form because it is the form that the body naturally produces. D3 is considered to be more stable and up to three times more potent than ergocalciferol.

But how does the body actually turn sunbeams into vitamin D in your bloodstream?

In Chapter 1, we looked at the short explanation of vitamin D synthesis created by the contact between UVB rays and the skin. When UVB rays interact with a pre-cholesterol within the top layer of the skin, they create a form of vitamin D that travels through the bloodstream to the liver and then to the kidneys where it becomes activated as a hormone and can be utilized by the body. Most importantly, vitamin D production depends on your exposure time and the strength of the sun's UVB rays. Below is a detailed explanation of this process.

How Your Skin Makes Vitamin D from the Sun: The Transformation of Vitamin D into Hormone D

- Step 1: UVB rays enter the top layer of skin (epidermis) and interacts with the cholesterol precursor (7-dehydrocholesterol) located within the epidermis to create pre-curser pre-vitamin D, which is then quickly converted within the skin to form pro-hormone vitamin D3 (cholecalciferol).

- Step 2: Vitamin D3 is released into the blood where it binds with a vitamin D–binding protein (VDBP) and is carried to the liver.

- Step 3: In the liver, vitamin D3 is hydroxylated through the action of the enzyme 25-hydroxylase to form the pre-hormone calcidiol, or 25-hydroxyvitamin D (25-D).

- Step 4: 25-D reenters the bloodstream where it binds to a VDBP and is taken up by the kidneys. In the kidneys, the hydroxylation process is repeated through the enzymatic action of 1-alpha-hydroxylase, transforming 25-D into the biologically active hormone called calcitriol, or 1,25-dihydroxyvitamin D (1,25-D).

- Step 5: Hormone 1,25-D enters the bloodstream, is bound to a VDBP, and hitches a ride to vitamin D receptor (VDR) sites throughout the body. Once this binding takes place, the VDR sites are activated.

- Step 6: Some of the 25-D goes directly to other tissues in the body where it converts to the active hormone 1,25-D. The process of other tissues being able to convert 25-D to the 1,25-D in glands is referred to as autocrine function. In other words, vitamin D is so important that other tissues of our body can convert the 25-D into the 1-25-D

Vitamin D from Skin Production, Food, and Supplements

While this chapter outlines the many benefits of obtaining vitamin D from the sun, it is also important to understand how the body processes the vitamin D that comes from food and supplements too. That fact is particularly important because, as pointed out in the beginning of this chapter, most people will need to supplement for vitamin D since they are not likely to get all of this crucial nutrient from the sun alone. Essentially, the steps for vitamin D synthesis within the body are similar whether it is obtained from the sun, food, or supplements. The main difference is that vitamin D from food and supplements enters the body through the mouth rather than the skin. After oral intake of vitamin D, it travels to the stomach and is absorbed through the small intestine. From the intestine, it is transported through the bloodstream to the liver and continues with the same steps given in the previous explanation of how the body makes vitamin D from the sun, starting with Step 2. For the oral intake of vitamin D, therefore, the steps for synthesis are:

- Step 1: Food or supplements containing vitamin D are taken orally and travel to the stomach before being absorbed by the small intestine.
- Steps 2 to 5: Vitamin D synthesis takes place in the same manner as it does for sun-produced vitamin D. (See illustration above.)

Keep in mind that the oral route can have many obstacles that reduce the amount of vitamin D that is absorbed. Vitamin D, like vitamins A, E, and K are fat-soluble vitamins. If a person has

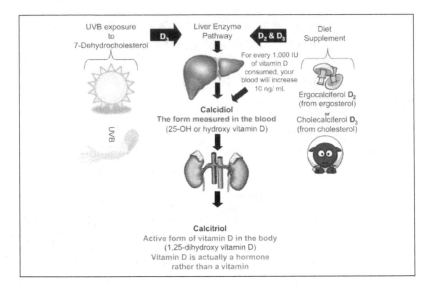

digestive problems, especially due to fat malabsorption, surgical removal of part of the intestines, or gastric bypass surgery, vitamin D may not be absorbed. This is yet another reason why getting some of your vitamin D from the sun is important.

The body's ability to synthesize vitamin D is a remarkable feat. And, as mentioned earlier, receptor sites for vitamin D are found throughout the body. We have just scratched the surface in terms of understanding the breadth of vitamin D's impact on our health. For one thing, we now know that vitamin D receptors are expressed in several types of immune cells, including white blood cells, T and B cells, and monocytes, where they support the immun e system. Cancer researchers are also finding that these same receptors are also involved in cell proliferation and differentiation, which has important medical implications since rampant proliferation of the wrong type of cells is at the core of the cancer process. Research is continuing to unravel this mystery, and someday we will likely be able to use some form of vitamin D to treat some types of cancer, or perhaps put it to work in other treatments that are still to be discovered.

Tapping the Sun for Vitamin D

Given the many established—and yet to be discovered—benefits of generating vitamin D from UVB rays, it is important to carefully weigh the risks and rewards of exposing your skin to the sun. This chapter has offered a great deal of information about how the body produces vitamin D from sun exposure, and perhaps you have gained some appreciation for the sun as a powerful source of health benefits. In the next chapter, you will learn about vitamin D deficiencies.

Key Points from Chapter 4 — Getting Vitamin D from the Sun

- The skin is the largest organ in the body

- Excessive exposure to these particular rays may also cause serious skin-damaging sunburns, that can lead to skin cancer

- UVB rays produce vitamin D3 and can burn the skin

- UVA rays tan the skin

- UVB and UVA cause cumulative skin damage

- UVA rays are strongest in summer, but are also strong all year round

- UVB rays do not penetrate glass. UVA rays do penetrate glass

- Access the UV Index in your area is through weather channels

Chapter 5

When the Sun Is Not Enough— Vitamin D Deficiencies

One of the most persistent myths about vitamin D is that most people can get a sufficient supply of it if you just spend ten or fifteen minutes in the sun a few times a week during the spring and summer. As with any myth, there is some truth to that statement—sunshine can produce vitamin D in your body. But as you now know from reading the previous chapters, you cannot make any vitamin D unless you specifically expose your body to the sun's UVB rays. Plus, the amount of vitamin D you can produce from the sun varies depending on your skin type as well as the latitude, altitude, time of day, season of the year, and other factors, including age.

As stated previously, most people cannot depend on the sun alone to produce the full amount of vitamin D that their bodies require. If you live near the equator, you could get most of your D from the sun. However, vitamin D deficiency is also a health hazard in sun-drenched Australia. The fact remains that most of us need dietary supplements to ensure a healthy tissue supply of this vital substance.

Nevertheless, many people continue to believe that if they are simply out in the sunshine from time to time, they will receive an adequate amount of D. That's what a middle-aged patient of mine thought when she came to see me about the cramps in her muscles and pain in her joints—pain that was so severe that she was unable to walk around the block. Although she often got a little afternoon sun while gardening once or twice a week, a blood test revealed that her vitamin D level was deficient. Over a two-month period, I advised her to up her vitamin D intake. Within four weeks, the muscle cramps and joint pain resolved, and she was able to walk pain free. Needless to say, she was thrilled.

A famous case attests to the fact that even someone who spends a great deal of time outdoors can still be deficient in vitamin D. While pursuing her dream of being an Olympic champion, Deena Kastor fractured a bone in her foot shortly after she began running a marathon at the 2008 games in Beijing. According to a report on her case in *Runner's World* magazine (in the December 2009 issue), a test revealed she was not absorbing enough calcium and phosphorus because her vitamin D levels were far too low. As a skin cancer survivor, she had been diligent about covering up and applying sunscreen. Therefore, even though she was out in the sun, she was unable to produce enough vitamin D through the limited amount of UVB rays that reached her skin. Once she was treated for vitamin D deficiency and began taking supplements for it, her levels stabilized, and she was able to resume her running career.

For these two women—my patient, described above, and Deena Kastor—the lack of vitamin D showed up in dramatic fashion. Symptoms of vitamin D deficiency, however, may not always be obvious. For instance, one of my outwardly healthy young patients complained of chronic colds and susceptibility to the flu—problems that were greatly reduced after increasing his intake of vitamin D. Further, those suffering from depression, heart disease, diabetes, and multiple types of cancer may also be vitamin D deficient, as researchers are beginning to discover.

Because research is ongoing (and more is needed), and because vitamin D deficiencies can sometimes be hidden, your doctor may not recognize the lack of D as one of your underlying health problems—nor conduct tests to check for this deficiency. Compounding this problem is the fact that many health professionals order the wrong type of vitamin D test for their patients, making an accurate diagnosis difficult. Chapter 6 offers details on proper tests and treatment for vitamin D deficiency.

Once you learn about all of the diseases and health problems that are linked to a vitamin D deficiency, you may be tempted to self-prescribe it and load up on supplements. Vitamin D, however, is not a cure-all, particularly in its oral supplement form. And, while it is rare, an extremely high-dose oral supplementation can lead to toxicity over time. Moreover, once a disease is present, less is known about the outcome of treating the disease with vitamin D. Vitamin D is also contraindicated for specific health conditions and in combination with certain medications that will be covered in Chapter 8.

To ensure that you are getting proper care and dosages for your individual case, keep in mind that illnesses and diseases are complex and often have multiple contributing factors. If you have a serious health condition, it is important for you to make sure that you and your health-care provider are knowledgeable about current research before you are treated with vitamin D.

Are You at Risk for Vitamin D Deficiency (Secondary Hyperparathyroidism)?

Now that you have learned a little about what can happen to the body when it does not have enough vitamin D, you may be wondering if you are vitamin D deficient. Or you may be concerned about the status of family members—a legitimate issue since infants and children have additional risk factors and special needs for vitamin D. Details on children and vitamin D are covered in Chapter 11. The risk factors below show that multiple environmental and health issues contribute to vitamin D deficiency. Prolonged vitamin D deficiency is also referred to as secondary hyperparathyroidism. Any of these risk factors can cause deficiency, and many of us will relate to more than one. For a definitive diagnosis, it is always best to test.

Risk Factors for Vitamin D Deficiency (Secondary Hyperparathyroidism)

- Living in northern or southern latitudes, especially above or below 37° latitude. Two cities above 37° are San Francisco, California, on the West Coast and Richmond, Virginia, on the East Coast. Remember: the farther away from the equator, the fewer UVB rays, especially in winter months. (See the latitude chart in Chapter 2 to view latitudes in both hemispheres.)
- Daily use of sunscreens: SPF 15 blocks 93 percent of UVB rays.
- Dark pigmented skin without enough sun exposure
- Living in foggy and/or smoggy areas: fog and smog reduce UVB rays.
- Indoor jobs or nightshift work that that results in minimal sun exposure.
- Living and working where tall buildings or trees block the sun
- Wearing clothing that covers the arms and legs
- Living in nursing homes, prisons, or other confined situations where sunlight is insufficient
- Aging: skin becomes less capable of producing vitamin D through sun exposure as we age.
- A strict vegetarian diet and especially vegans, are more at risk since their diet is often devoid of vitamin D.
- An extremely low-fat diet, since vitamin D is fat soluble
- Intestinal fat malabsorption, including Ulcerative colitis, Crohn's disease, celiac disease, or cystic fibrosis
- Surgical removal of part or all of the small intestine or stomach
- Cushing's syndrome, a condition of the adrenal glands

- Hyperthyroidism or hypothyroidism. Primary Hyperparathyroidism—this is not the same as secondary hyperparathyroidism. This is covered in detail in Chapter 6
- Obesity: people who are obese often need to take a higher dose of vitamin D in order to increase their blood level.
- Kidney, liver, or gallbladder disease
- Alcoholism
- Hyperparathyroidism: Not enough exposure to vitamin D–producing UVB rays that results in a low blood calcium, and an increase in circulating parathyroid hormone, which results in bone breakdown and a known secondary risk factor for osteoporosis.
- Excessive caffeine or salt intake
- Diets high in processed foods
- Cigarette smoking: smoking has been shown to decrease the blood level of 25-D and 1,25-D.
- Medications, including over-the-counter medicines, can interfere with vitamin D absorption and synthesis. (See Chapter 8 for a list of known medications that interfere with vitamin D.)

The risk factors for vitamin D deficiency can alert you to potential problems and the need for testing and possible treatment. The list of illnesses involving or associated with vitamin D deficiency is extensive and, in some cases, quite surprising. Few other nutrients affect so many of the body's systems and functions, and this is because in its active form, vitamin D is a hormone with receptor sites throughout the body and virtually every gland. In recent years, research on vitamin D has skyrocketed and broadened to include thousands of studies investigating the unique and wide array of biological functions of the active vitamin D hormone.

As we learn more about D deficiency, new hope emerges for the potential of vitamin D treatments for specific conditions. The next section offers an overview of this research and some of the conditions associated with deficiency. It is worth a reminder here, however, that vitamin D is not a cure-all. In fact, vitamin D should be part of an overall nutritional program to make sure other nutrients that work with vitamin D such as vitamin K2 and magnesium are also present in the diet. You will learn more about these nutrients in chapter 6.

Treating the conditions associated with vitamin D deficiency is an area of research still evolving. Recovery from any illness is facilitated by a healthy lifestyle that may include safe sun exposure, vitamin D supplementation (see Chapter 8), an appropriate level of exercise, and a diet consistently high in antioxidants that includes vegetables, fruits, and omega 3 oils, and low in processed carbohydrates.

Vitamin D Deficiency and Disease Conditions

We know that vitamin D is essential for our well-being, as the evidence linking vitamin D deficiency to bone health and many forms of cancer is now overwhelming. Therefore, it is very important to maintain a healthy vitamin D status, meaning that your level is high enough to afford you the many benefits of this health-promoting hormone.

How is it possible that vitamin D impacts so many bodily functions? Virtually every tissue type in your body has receptors for vitamin D, meaning that they all require vitamin D for proper functioning. So, a deficiency of vitamin D can have far-reaching health consequences.

The early symptoms of vitamin D deficiency are common and often subtle it in the early stages. Some symptoms such as aches and pains can be easily dismissed because there are many things that can cause them. Some of these symptoms include muscle weakness, constant respiratory problems, depression, chronic infections, chronic pain, tiredness, muscle cramps (especially the calf muscle), reduced endurance, depression, crankiness, and increased PMS symptoms.

Active vitamin D works by entering cells and attaching to a protein called the vitamin D receptor, located in the nucleus of cells where the genetic material is located. This combination of calcitriol and its receptor stimulates the cell to make proteins that regulate the way the body works.

NOTE: Conditions due to vitamin D deficiency are associated with a prolonged deficiency. In other words, an inadequate amount may not result in rickets or osteomalacia (adult rickets), while a severe long-term deficiency can result in these serious conditions.

Joint, Muscle, Skeletal

Vitamin D is instrumental for our entire structural system. Vitamin D receptors are in our joints, structural muscles, and bones.

- Osteoporosis (*osteo* = bone; *por* = porous; *osis* = condition of). In Chapter 4, we learned how vitamin D is essential for building and maintaining a healthy skeletal system throughout life. The condition of osteoporosis is a growing problem around the world. If you ask people what the most important nutrient for bone health is, the most common answer is likely to be calcium. However, we also need vitamin D to make sure our dietary calcium and phosphorus is absorbed. Numerous studies link vitamin D deficiency to low bone mineral density (BMD). This is why it is so important for those who have been diagnosed with osteoporosis, both men and women, to be testing for their vitamin D status.

If BMD is low, there is a reason. Very often diet and lifestyle choices are strong contributors to the development of weakened bones, as are family genetics. I firmly believe that nutritional and lifestyle counseling should be at the top of health-care providers' list of suggestions to help patients achieve their healthiest possible bone quality and bone density.

Unfortunately, medications are routinely offered to patients with little attempt to diagnose and to correct the underlying problem of vitamin D deficiency or other conditions. Studies show that reversing vitamin D deficiency along with exercising and maintaining good nutrition can, in some cases, stabilize bone loss or produce a gain in bone density.

Women, who are most at risk of developing osteoporosis, can lose up to 20 percent of their BMD, beginning just before menopause and continuing the five to seven years following it. Some studies have shown that estrogen and vitamin D have a synergistic effect on bone.

Estrogen primarily inhibits osteoclastic activity, the cells that break down bone, while vitamin D primarily impacts osteoblasts (OB), the cells that increase bone growth. The interaction of vitamin D and osteoblasts is complicated, and what we know for sure is that vitamin D receptors are integrated in osteoblast cells. Some studies point to concerns that when the vitamin D blood level is too high, it may result in increased bone resorption. In chapter 6, you will learn about the vitamin D target amount in the serum. The bottom line is that a healthy vitamin D status is important to maintain always, and especially during menopausal years for women.

As an aside, frozen shoulder is common in women who are going through menopause. I have seen many patients with it in my practice, sometimes affecting both shoulders. My theory is that it may be the result of a vitamin D deficiency along with declining estrogen. Both have been shown to impact joint health.

- Osteomalacia (*osteo* = bone; *malacia* = wasting): Osteomalacia is often referred to as "adult rickets." This condition is marked by a softening of the bones, most often caused by severe and prolonged vitamin D deficiency. Lab results of patients having osteomalacia will show vitamin D deficiency that results in low calcium in the blood, thus robbing the bones of this vital nutrient. Osteomalacia is a known cause of persistent, nonspecific musculoskeletal pain. In fact, pressing a bone in the forearm or sternum often results in a significant pain response.

- Rickets: Rickets is a disease that often begins in the womb or early childhood before bones have fully developed. Its primary cause is vitamin D deficiency that also leads to calcium deficiency during crucial bone development in childhood. Infants with rickets display delayed crawling, sitting, and standing. Prolonged deficiency produces weak bones that are too soft to support the weight of the body, resulting in bowed legs, spinal curvature, and lack of growth in the body's long bones.

In today's world, one of the known risk factors for the development of rickets is due to expectant mothers who are vitamin D deficient during pregnancy and lactation; in these cases, studies have shown that vitamin D is low in mother's milk. As children develope and grow, in today's world, many spend most of their day time hours indoors. In fact, in most schools today, physical education classes have been cut from the curriculum.

Other symptoms include extreme muscle cramping and, in some cases, lack of mental development. In the 1930s, after discovering vitamin D could cure rickets, milk and other foods were fortified with vitamin D, and rickets was almost totally eradicated. Now, however, cases of rickets are reappearing with disturbing frequency. If this disfiguring and debilitating disease is to be successfully combated, nutritional attention must be directed to children and adolescents, as around 80 percent of our lifetime bone mass is laid down by the age of eighteen.

- Unexplained Muscle and Joint Pain: In a study of 150 children and adults with unexplained muscle and bone pain, almost all were found to be vitamin D deficient. The deficiency was pervasive: all of the African Americans, East Africans, Hispanics, and Native Americans who participated in the study were deficient, as were all of the patients under the age of thirty. From this we can see that it is crucial to the health of those in the above-mentioned ethnic groups, as well as for all children and adolescents, that vitamin D levels be ascertained as part of considering an overall health regimen, particularly in the presence of unexplained muscle and joint pain.

  Hypothyroidism and fibromyalgia are two diagnoses with the same symptoms (muscle and joint pain) as vitamin D deficiency. Vitamin D testing would be useful in these cases.

- Sarcopenia, Muscle Wasting: The loss of muscle strength is often seen in older adults and has many causes, including the loss of hormones and vitamin D. Vitamin D deficiency is one suggested component of muscle loss. Advanced osteoporosis is often coupled with sarcopenia.

- Osteoarthritis (*osteo* = bone; *arth* = joint; *itis* = inflammation) also referred to as degenerative joint disease (DJD):

Osteoarthrosis is a common "wear and tear" disease that occurs when the cartilage that serves as a cushion in the joints deteriorates. This condition can affect any joint but is most common in knees, hands, hips, and spine. When the joint is inflamed, osteoarthrosis is then termed *osteoarthritis* (OA). OA can be acute or chronic.

There can be a genetic propensity regarding the development of OA and DJD. However, early joint deterioration most often arises in joints that have endured significant injuries. Joints that have sustained repetitive trauma from work activities, heavy lifting, or sport activities that involve substantial joint use or high impact over time can also result in joint deterioration.

Several studies have shown that vitamin D provides a protective benefit that reduces cartilage breakdown. One thirty-month study conducted in 2004 followed 221 elderly patients with osteoarthritis of the knee. Those who were shown to be deficient in vitamin D were given 800 IU of vitamin D daily. Of the patients whose low blood level of vitamin D showed improvement, disability scores were improved.

■ Fibromyalgia (*fibro* = fibrous tissue; *my* = muscle; *algia* = pain): The hallmark symptoms of fibromyalgia are chronic muscular pain, fatigue, headaches, and irritable bowel. Many conditions have similar symptoms, including vitamin D deficiency, which can be the root cause of unresolved muscle and joint pain. Patients who are diagnosed with fibromyalgia should be tested for vitamin D deficiency.

■ Poor Tooth Development and Cavities (periodontal disease and dental caries): Vitamin D deficiency during pregnancy can cause enamel hypoplasia of primary teeth. Teeth require vitamin D to develop and remain strong. Teeth are made of minerals like calcium and phosphate. When the tooth structure is weak, tooth decay is more common, and poor tooth quality can also result in teeth that fracture (crack) more easily. While studies are inconclusive, many point to a connection between oral health and vitamin D. Receding gums can be the result of bone loss in the bones of the jaw, which is more common starting in middle age. Teeth that loosen could be the result of advanced osteoporosis. However, loose teeth can also be the result of a local infection.

■ Fingernail Issues: Fingernails are composed of laminated layers of a protein called keratin, which is also found in hair and skin. Many health conditions and nutrient deficiencies can lead to fingernails that are weak or brittle. Vitamin D deficiency that results in low blood calcium may result in flimsy nails. Once I corrected my own vitamin D deficiency, my flimsy nails thickened, likely due to the increase of calcium absorption.

■ Hair Issues: Vitamin D stimulates hair follicles to grow. Vitamin D deficiency is a suggested link to alopecia areata, an autoimmune condition that causes patchy hair loss. Some studies show that women experiencing other forms of hair loss have much lower levels of vitamin D.

■ Hearing Loss (otosclerosis): Otosclerosis is the number one cause of hearing loss. Research implicates vitamin D deficiency as a potential cause in some cases of otosclerosis, the term for abnormal bone growth in the middle ear, in which the consistency of the sound-conducting bones of the ear changes from hard, mineralized bone to spongy, immature bone tissue.

Otosclerosis is the leading cause of middle ear hearing loss in young adults, affecting about 10 percent of the population of the United States. Even though otosclerosis has a strong familial origin, vitamin D deficiency may, in fact, trigger its development in some cases.

Cancer

Although randomized clinical trial data are still lacking, several epidemiological, clinical, preclinical, and in vitro experimental data strongly suggest vitamin D prevents certain cancers and ultimately may be used to treat some forms of cancer.

In studies of cancer cells and of tumors in mice, vitamin D has been found to perform several activities that might slow or prevent the development of cancer, including promoting cellular differentiation, decreasing cancer cell growth, stimulating cell death (apoptosis), and reducing tumor blood vessel formation (angiogenesis). The National Institute of Health states that "strong biological and mechanistic bases indicate that vitamin D plays a role in the prevention of colon, prostate, and breast cancers."

One of the key players in vitamin D cancer research is William B. Grant, PhD. I have interviewed Dr. Grant on several occasions. When we spoke, he said that more than twenty-five cancers have been linked to vitamin D deficiency. "Results for breast and colorectal cancer satisfy the criteria best, but there is also good evidence that other cancers do as well, including bladder, esophageal, gallbladder, gastric, ovarian, rectal, renal, and uterine corpus cancer, as well as Hodgkin's and non-Hodgkin's lymphoma. Several cancers have mixed findings with respect to UVB and/or vitamin D, including pancreatic and prostate cancer and melanoma."

At the same time that vitamin D is emerging as a potential treatment for some forms of cancer, other studies question earlier findings and suggest that some cancers may worsen in the presence of higher vitamin D blood levels. Widely diverging opinions and disparate findings within the scientific community are evidence of vitamin D's emergence as a key element to many aspects of our health. Stay tuned.

Heart Health

The following is an excerpt from Johns Hopkins' website: "A growing number of studies point to vitamin D deficiency as a risk factor for heart attacks, congestive heart failure, peripheral arterial disease (PAD), strokes, and the conditions associated with cardiovascular disease, such as high blood pressure and diabetes."

Dr. Erin Michos, Assistant Professor of Medicine at Johns Hopkins Hospital in the Division of Cardiology, has examined and contributed a great deal of data on vitamin D deficiency and the heart, including a study published in the Archives of Internal Medicine.

The role of vitamin D supplementation in the management of cardiovascular disease remains to be established.

- Coronary Heart Disease (CHD): Higher vitamin D levels may lower the risk of CHD. In a 2006 study, patients with CHD showed elevated inflammatory markers. After receiving 2,000 IU of vitamin D daily for nine months, they showed a significant suppression of pro-inflammatory markers and an increase in anti-inflammatory markers. The arteries of those whose inflammation markers were elevated may be subject to increased amounts of plaque building up in the arteries, including coronary arteries, leaving these patients vulnerable to heart attack or stroke. Vitamin D's anti-inflammatory action in the arteries implies that vitamin D has a protective role in heart and artery health.
- Atherosclerosis or Peripheral Artery Disease (*athero* = artery; *scler* = hardening; *osis* = condition of): Known as PAD, this disease is characterized by blood vessels outside the heart

and brain that accumulate enough plaque buildup to restrict blood flow. The same protective mechanism mentioned above for coronary arteries applies to peripheral arteries too. Over time, arteries that carry blood to the legs, arms, stomach, or kidneys build up plaque and consequently narrow, resulting in restricted blood flow. Those afflicted with PAD often have difficulty walking due to pain. Studies link vitamin D deficiency as one potential cause of PAD, since vitamin D has an anti-inflammatory action on blood vessels.

- Hypertension (elevated blood pressure): Studies have demonstrated a possible link between hypertension and vitamin D deficiency. The Mayo Clinic reports the following: "Low levels of vitamin D may play a role in the development of high blood pressure. It has been noted that blood pressure is often elevated under the following conditions: during the winter season, at a further distance from the equator, and in individuals with dark skin pigmentation (all of which are associated with lower production of vitamin D via sunlight). However, evidence is not clear, and a comparison with more proven methods to reduce blood pressure has not been conducted."

  A 2017 study concluded, "Significant race/ethnic and gender differences exist in the association of vitamin D and systolic blood pressure. Odds for hypertension are reduced significantly at higher vitamin D levels, but this benefit plateaus at very high vitamin D levels."

Menopause

Some women report an array of difficult, even debilitating, symptoms as they enter menopause, including mood swings, hot flashes, night sweats, heart palpitations, weight gain, diminished or increased libido, and bone loss. Extreme symptoms can be exacerbated by high stress, lack of exercise, poor diet, alcohol, and tobacco use. Vitamin D deficiency can increase the severity of symptoms in several ways, including a decrease in calcium absorption. Likewise, vitamin D has a balancing effect on female hormones, and for some, it may help diminish menopause discomfort.

Premenstrual Syndrome (PMS)

Researchers at the University of British Columbia found that the symptoms associated with PMS—depression, irritability, fatigue, and oversleeping—lessened in the summer and intensified during winter months.

A 2016 randomized controlled trial discovered that vitamin D supplementation significantly reduced anxiety, irritability, and sadness in young women with concomitant mood disorders linked to PMS. PMS cramping could also easily be connected to vitamin D deficiency resulting in low-serum calcium. Calcium has been shown to reduce symptoms of PMS symptoms.

Furthermore, a 2018 study concluded, "Thorough assessment of vitamin D deficiency/insufficiency is required among patients with menstrual disorders, especially those overweight and obese. Early screening and VD supplementation in women with estrogen-dependent disorders may become a part of routine management in order to optimize endocrine health."

Infertility and Ovulation: Issues for Men and Women

Animal studies show that vitamin D deficiency negatively affects ovulation and the menstrual cycle. Research has shown that vitamin D plays a regulatory role in reproductive physiology. Since vitamin D receptors and enzymes are expressed in the ovaries, placenta, testis, and male reproductive tract, researchers hypothesized that vitamin D may act locally to mediate the effects on the reproductive system.

Endometriosis

Several studies have shown a link between vitamin D deficiency and endometriosis. Low levels of vitamin D appear to be connected both to endometriosis onset and to its severity, researchers said in a study that found that women with the lowest blood concentrations of the vitamin also had the largest ovarian endometrioma, or ovarian cysts. The study, "Ovarian Endometriosis and Vitamin D Serum Levels," was published in *Gynecological Endocrinology*. Its findings suggest that vitamin D supplements could be a safe and low-cost therapeutic approach, since vitamin D can modulate inflammation and proliferation in endometriotic cells.

Endometriosis seems to result from a combination of genetic, hormonal, immunological, and environmental factors. Yet, inflammation processes play an important role in the development and progression of the disease. Vitamin D is known to reduce inflammatory responses, and it has been shown to have regulating effects on the immune system. The potential role of vitamin D in immune diseases is drawing increased interest, and previous studies have found anti-inflammatory effects in diseases such as rheumatoid arthritis and psoriasis, and decreased tumor growth in cancers.

Women with endometriosis tend to have lower vitamin D levels compared to the general female population, higher levels of which seem to be associated with a lower risk of getting the disease, according to studies.

Polycystic Ovary Syndrome (PCOS)

According to findings published in the *Journal of Clinical Endocrinology & Metabolism*, vitamin D deficiency in PCOS patients who have undergone fertility treatment with ovarian stimulation is associated with a diminished rate of ovulation and pregnancy and a lower chance of a live birth.

Hypothyroidism (low thyroid function)

Women are far more likely than men to develop hypothyroidism. Most commonly, low thyroid function develops during pregnancy and menopause, when estrogen and progesterone levels are imbalanced or diminishing. The primary cause of hypothyroidism is the autoimmune disease Hashimoto's thyroiditis (inflammation of the thyroid), which is diagnosed by an elevation of thyroid antibodies (TPO) and typically elevated thyroid stimulating hormone (TSH).

One study found that the patients with autoimmune thyroid disease had vitamin D3 levels that were significantly lower than the controls. And, interestingly, almost 82 percent of the autoimmune thyroid disease patients had low vitamin D. The patients who had especially high TPO antibodies—above 1,300—showed *significantly lower* vitamin D3 levels.

Headaches and Migraines

Migraines are a severe form of headache that can be debilitating for many people and are more common in women than in men. Studies have shown a correlation between migraines and the menstrual cycle.

Research shows that vitamin D deficiency is common in patients with headaches and chronic migraine. During a presentation at an American Headache Society meeting, Dr. Ryan Wheeler explained that over 40 percent of patients with chronic headaches and migraines were vitamin D deficient.

Mental Health

Some studies have implicated *vitamin D deficiency* to a wide range of psychiatric illnesses and it is an emerging area of interest for researchers. Following are some of the conditions that have a potential connection with prolonged vitamin D deficiency.

- Depression: A variety of nutritional deficiencies can play a large role in chronic depression. While studies remain unclear, vitamin D deficiency is a likely player in depression. Psychiatrist John Cannell of the Vitamin D Council writes, "Evidence exists that major depression is associated with low vitamin D levels and that depression has increased in the last century as vitamin D levels have surely fallen. Evidence exists that depression is associated with heart disease, hypertension, diabetes, rheumatoid arthritis, cancer, and low bone mineral density, all illnesses thought to be caused, in part, by vitamin D deficiency. Finally, vitamin D has profound effects on the brain including the neurotransmitters involved in major depression."

- Anxiety: In the April 2007 *Journal of Clinical Rheumatology* a study reported an association of anxiety in those diagnosed with fibromyalgia. This particular group (those with fibromyalgia who reported having anxiety) also had vitamin D deficiency. Since anxiety can also be the result of adrenal, thyroid, and sex hormone imbalances, it is not a far stretch to conclude that some people with anxiety may benefit from vitamin D supplementation. Also, the decreased calcium absorption associated with vitamin D deficiency is critical for the nervous system and has a calming effect.

- Psychosis—Schizophrenia: Vitamin D deficiency during gestation may increase the risk of schizophrenia. Vitamin D researcher Dr. Darryl Eyles states it this way: "Undeniably, low maternal vitamin D affects the way the brain develops."

  Furthermore, a diagnosis of schizophrenia is more prevalent in African American children than in Caucasian children. Pregnant women with dark skin are especially at risk for vitamin D deficiency. As mentioned in Chapter 3, dark skin may require as much as six to twelve times more UVB rays to produce the same amount of vitamin D as what is required for light skin. Low vitamin D in African Americans could be one of the reasons psychoses is higher in this particular group.

A 2004 Finnish study concluded, "Vitamin D supplementation during the first year of life is associated with a reduced risk of schizophrenia in males. Preventing hypovitaminosis D during early life may reduce the incidence of schizophrenia."

■ Insomnia: For people suffering serious insomnia, vitamin D deficiency should always be ruled out, as vitamin D directly affects calcium homeostasis (calcium metabolism: the mechanism by which the body maintains adequate calcium levels). Calcium has a calming effect on the body. Some cases of insomnia respond well to an increase of vitamin D. Also, vitamin D is associated with brain chemistry, thyroid, and sex hormone imbalances. There seems to be an ongoing theme here in that, as with previous deficiency syndromes, vitamin D may play a key role.

Another cause of insomnia involves light and has to do with how natural sunlight affects circadian rhythms. When these rhythms are significantly disturbed it can impair one's ability to sleep well.

(NOTE: In Chapter 12, you will learn more about how sunlight itself impacts insomnia.)

Body Weight

■ Weight Loss/Gain: Observational studies of farm animals that do not receive sunlight show that they have a higher percentage of body fat compared to animals exposed to sunlight. One study exposed animals to UVB rays, thus increasing the animal's vitamin D levels, and noted that they lost weight. This may be explained by vitamin D's stimulation of thyroid function, which leads to increased production of thyroid hormones that in turn regulate metabolism. When metabolism is stimulated, calories burn more efficiently. One symptom of low thyroid function (hypothyroidism) is weight gain.

■ Obesity: It is well established that vitamin D is low in people who are obese. This is because vitamin D is a fat-soluble vitamin, and it is stored in fat cells. Excess fat locks up available vitamin D, whereas a normal-weight person recycles their fat-releasing vitamin D into their bloodstream. According to vitamin D researcher Michael Holick, obese people need two to three times the amount of vitamin D as a normal-weight person needs to maintain a healthy vitamin D level.

Autoimmune Diseases and Vitamin D

An autoimmune disease is one in which the body produces antibodies that attack its own tissues, leading to the deterioration and, in some cases, the destruction of such tissue. Immune system disorders cause abnormally low activity or overactivity of the immune system. In cases of immune system overactivity, the body attacks and damages its own tissues (autoimmune diseases). Immune deficiency diseases decrease the body's ability to fight invaders, causing vulnerability to infections.

An autoimmune disease is characterized as the body "attacking" itself because normally, antibodies and lymphocytes keep us healthy by fighting alien substances including bacteria and viruses. Autoimmune diseases cause antibodies and lymphocytes to attack normal tissue as if it were foreign.

Epidemiologists have shown that the prevalence of autoimmune diseases is much lower in tropical regions where there is ample sunshine and, thus, vitamin D. Vitamin D is not only a powerful hormone; it also acts as an antioxidant that supports and stimulates the immune system. However, some autoimmune diseases will worsen if the immune system is stimulated. In certain autoimmune conditions, vitamin D is contraindicated or must be monitored carefully to manage the autoimmune disease. Anyone suffering with an autoimmune disorder should work with a specialist who is steeped in nutrition and vitamin D supplementation.

Systemic lupus erythematosus (SLE)

SLE is eight times more common in women than men. The causes of SLE are unknown. However, heredity, viruses, ultraviolet light, and certain medications may all play a role. SLE can cause disease of the skin, heart, lungs, kidneys, joints, and nervous system. When only the skin is involved, the condition is called discoid lupus. When internal organs are involved, the condition is called systemic lupus erythematosus (SLE).

The conclusion of a 2018 study regarding SLE reported that lower levels of vitamin D are associated with higher disease activity rates. Therefore, it is important to evaluate vitamin D supplementation in patients with SLE as part of the treatment, especially when it includes the use of steroids.

Inflammatory Bowel Disease

The most common inflammatory bowel diseases (IBD) conditions are Crohn's disease and ulcerative colitis. These conditions may be either autoimmune disease or autoimmune-mediated diseases and have been associated with vitamin D deficiency. Ulcerative colitis affects the large intestine, while Crohn's disease most commonly affects the small intestine. People with these conditions typically have lower vitamin D levels due to malabsorption of vitamin D. In addition, people with IBD are often treated with prednisone, which depletes vitamin D.

An interesting Scandinavian study randomized people with Crohn's disease in remission to vitamin D or placebo. At the end of the year, there was a tendency toward lower rates of relapse in people treated with vitamin D compared with placebo. The relapse rate in the vitamin D arm was 13percent, compared with 29 percent in patients who received placebo, suggesting that vitamin D may play a role in preventing relapse.

Diabetes and Insulin Resistance

Insulin is a hormone that converts sugar, starches, and other food into the energy that fuels our body. It works by "unlocking" the cells of the body, allowing glucose to enter and then fuel the cells. If the body fails to produce insulin, Type 1 (diabetes mellitus) results. Only about 5 to 10 percent of Americans who are diagnosed with diabetes have Type 1, which is an autoimmune disorder.

Type 2 diabetes refers to the condition in which the body does produce insulin but is unable to use it properly. This is referred to as insulin resistance. Most Americans who are diagnosed with diabetes have Type 2 diabetes. Vitamin D plays a pivotal role in cellular health and metabolism, and it is critical to make sure vitamin D status is sufficient in diabetics. Vitamin D is believed to help improve the body's sensitivity to insulin and thus reduce the risk of insulin resistance, which is often a precursor to Type 2 diabetes.

Type 1 diabetes is a hereditary condition. However, studies suggest a role for vitamin D in the pathogenesis and prevention of Type 1 diabetes. The active hormone vitamin D (1,25-D) has been shown to prevent Type 1 diabetes in animal models. Perhaps vitamin D deficiency during pregnancy or during early childhood may precipitate the onset of Type 1 diabetes.

Multiple Sclerosis

Epidemiologic evidence regarding a link between multiple sclerosis (MS) and vitamin D deficiency is strong. The incidence of MS is significantly higher the farther away from the equator one lives. One study showed that women with higher vitamin D blood levels were 40 percent less likely to develop MS. Treatment of MS using vitamin D is showing promise.

Parkinson's Disease (PD)

The following statement is credited to the Rutgers Cancer Institute of New Jersey: "We hypothesize, based upon several lines of evidence, that documented chronically inadequate vitamin D intake in the United States, particularly in the northern states and particularly in the elderly, is a significant factor in the pathogenesis of PD."

Rheumatoid Arthritis (RA)

Several studies have linked vitamin D deficiency with RA. The Women's Health Study (WHS) consisted of following thirty thousand female subjects aged fifty-five to sixty-nine for an eleven-year period. One hundred fifty-two of these women developed RA. Women who ingested less than a meager 200 IU of vitamin D daily were 33 percent more likely to develop this debilitating autoimmune condition than those who consumed more than 200 IU.

Following is a statement on this disease from the National Institutes of Health website: "Reduced vitamin D intake has been linked to increased susceptibility to the development of rheumatoid arthritis (RA) and vitamin D deficiency has been found to be associated with disease activity in patients with RA."

Psoriasis

Psoriasis is an autoimmune condition that results in overproduction of skin cells, causing the skin to scale and slough. It is a condition characterized by patches of irritated, flaky skin that usually appear on the elbows and knees and across the trunk, and it tends to be especially active in winter. New research may help explain why. Scientists in Italy found that people with psoriasis also suffer from vitamin D deficiency. "We speculated that vitamin D might be low in psoriasis patients, but this is the first good study that substantiates it," says Dr. Suzanne Olbricht, an associate professor of dermatology at Harvard Medical School.

Henry Lim, MD, chief of dermatology at Detroit's Henry Ford Hospital, said that UVB light therapy is an effective treatment for about 70 percent of patients, and vitamin D creams improve symptoms in about 50 to 60 percent of patients with mild psoriasis. You will learn more about UV light treatments in Chapter 11.

Eczema

At least a dozen studies have found that both children and adults with *eczema* are more likely to have low levels of *vitamin D*. Research has also found that people who have *eczema* and low levels of *vitamin D* are more likely to get infections on their skin. Studies suggest that daily vitamin D supplementation might help children with eczema that gets worse in the winter. When eczema, a chronic inflammatory skin disorder, flares up in the winter it's known as winter-related atopic dermatitis.

Eczema is an inflammation of the skin. Once diagnosed, patients are often told that it is a genetic disorder and that they will likely have it off and on for the rest of their lives. Even though eczema is not considered a vitamin D deficiency per se, some people recover with ultraviolet light (UVB and UVA) treatment. If you have eczema, consider "feeding" your skin with a nutritious diet that includes vitamin D, probiotics (friendly intestinal bacteria), and evening primrose oil (taking 500 mg twice a day orally). Topical evening primrose oil has been helpful for some. Food allergies are a common feature of eczema outbreaks.

As an aside, I myself was plagued with eczema from my childhood through early adulthood. I always had eczema during the winter. In my early twenties, I worked on a kibbutz in Israel that was located in the desert. My eczema resolved and has never returned.

Digestive Disorders

Any condition that impairs absorption of nutrients or fat will affect the absorption of vitamin D, a fat-soluble vitamin. Some conditions that impair absorption of nutrients or fat include malabsorption syndrome, irritable bowel syndrome (IBS), and inflammatory bowel diseases such as Crohn's disease and ulcerative colitis. Symptoms of digestive disorders are sometimes obvious and include burping, excessive gas, bloating, loose stools, or constipation. Less obvious symptoms include skin rashes and fatigue. Digestive disorders can often be diagnosed and healed if your doctor is tuned in to natural healing options.

Low vitamin D status is common among the irritable bowel syndrome (IBS) population and merits assessment. An inverse correlation between serum vitamin D and IBS symptom severity is suggested and vitamin D interventions may benefit symptoms.

Intestinal Surgery Including Bypass

People who have had surgical removal of any part of the small intestine or stomach must be monitored for vitamin deficiencies, including a vitamin D deficiency. Disease processes, such as osteoporosis, that are the result of deficiencies take time to develop, so regular monitoring of vitamin D levels is strongly recommended, at least twice yearly. Interestingly, specific areas of the small intestine absorb vitamin D and calcium.

- Calcium and Vitamin D: Multiple reports discuss deficiencies of calcium and vitamin D and hyperparathyroidism in patients who have had recent gastric bypass surgery. Aggressive supplementation of calcium and vitamin D has been recommended around the time of the operation to combat these adverse effects. See Chapter 7 for more information about testing the above-mentioned nutrients.

Infectious Diseases

- Tuberculosis: Low vitamin D levels were associated with a five-fold increased risk for progression to tuberculosis. Deficiency of vitamin D (25-hydroxycholecalciferol) has long been implicated in activation of tuberculosis (TB). Serum levels of vitamin D in TB patients are lower than in healthy controls. However, treatment with high doses of vitamin D did not show significant benefit regarding treating TB.

Defy Deficiencies

This chapter focused on a partial list of diseases and other medical conditions that have been linked to vitamin D deficiency. To avoid these health problems, it is important to make sure that you and your family are getting enough vitamin D from sensible sun exposure, from food sources, and, when necessary, from vitamin D supplementation. If you are not getting enough vitamin D, the following chapter will guide you in vitamin D testing and in ways to make sure your vitamin D level is optimal.

Key Points from Chapter 5 — When the Sun Is Not Enough—Vitamin D Deficiencies

■ Vitamin D deficiencies are common, especially in higher or lower latitudes

■ Vitamin D deficiency is also called secondary hyperparathyroidism

■ An SPF 15 sunscreen blocks 93 percent of UVB rays

■ The early symptoms of vitamin D deficiency are often subtle

■ Some early symptoms of vitamin D deficiency such as aches and pains can be easily dismissed

■ Chronic infections, depression, and muscle cramps can be due to vitamin D deficiency

Chapter 6

Vitamin D Testing and Associated Tests

You may think that taking high doses of vitamin D is a good idea based on what you have heard or read. Unless you have your vitamin D tested, you cannot be sure how much vitamin D you have on board or how much you might need to take as a supplement. Vitamin D supplementation should not be taken lightly. There are some health conditions where vitamin D supplementation is contraindicated, which you will learn about in Chapter 8. However, there are two conditions, in particular, that may be overlooked by you or your health-care provider before implementing vitamin D supplementation. These are hypercalcemia (elevated blood calcium) and hypercalciuria (elevated urinary output of calcium).

The two conditions mentioned above are always listed as contraindications, but how many doctors order these tests, and how many laypeople know about them before taking vitamin D supplements? I have seen too many patients over the years who have supplemented with high doses of vitamin D when it was contraindicated. Primary hyperparathyroidism (pHPD) is one common condition that results in elevated blood calcium that you will learn more about later in this chapter.

My previous book was about osteoporosis. Over the years, I have found that many doctors do not understand the connection between the parathyroid glands, serum calcium, vitamin D and osteoporosis. Because of this, patients can be prescribed inappropriate vitamin D supplementation. Understanding the interaction between calcium, vitamin D, and the parathyroid glands is what you will learn about in the following sections.

Next you will learn about vitamin D testing, and then the important tests that should be considered in addition to the vitamin D test. You will also learn about how vitamin D works with other hormones to regulate calcium (homeostasis) so that you can make informed decisions regarding supplementing with vitamin D.

An important side note to vitamin D testing is that in 2018 the U.S. Preventive Services Task Force draft recommendation stated there is insufficient evidence that routine screening is effective. They concluded that further studies are necessary to assess the need for screening the population for vitamin D deficiency. In my opinion, vitamin D testing is important if one has risk factors for vitamin D deficiency.

So, can you take vitamin D without testing, and if so, how much is safe? Is testing important and is it reliable? Are there other tests that should be ordered along with vitamin D testing? These are the questions that we will work through in this chapter and Chapter 7. For now, you will learn about the two vitamin D tests that can be ordered by your doctor and some home test kits.

Vitamin D Testing— How to Know if You are Low

There are two main tests used to measure vitamin D level in the blood. The names of these tests are similar, so sometimes health professionals and patients can be confused about which test is best to assess vitamin D status. These tests are the 25-D (25, hydroxy-vitamin D) test and the 1,25-D test (1,25 dihydroxy-vitamin D). The 25-D test is the correct test to order to determine your vitamin D status.

The 25-D test represents the vitamin D that you have obtained from all sources including: the sun, food and supplements. If you remember, we learned about the conversion of vitamin D to 25 hydroxy-vitamin D (25-D). Vitamin D undergoes a conversion (hydroxylation) in the liver. When it reenters the blood stream, it is in the form of 25-D. It is then primarily transported to the kidneys, where it is converted to the active hormone, 1,25-D (calcitriol). The important thing to remember is this: the 1,25-D test *does not* assess vitamin D status.

Note: The 25-D and the 1,25-D test can include sources from D2 and D3. On the report it would be listed as total that includes both D2 and D3 combined and then would show how much D2 and D3 is in the bloodstream.

NOTE: At times, it is important to know the level of the 1,25-D hormone for specific diagnostic purposes such as osteoporosis or kidney disease.

Most notably the 1-25D test can be elevated when 25-D is low. At the same time, the parathyroid test (PTH-Intact) may also be elevated. When these findings are present with a LOW serum calcium, this finding is known as secondary hyperparathyroidism due to vitamin D deficiency. When vitamin D is low, typically serum calcium is low or on the low end of normal. And vitamin D deficiency NEVER results in an elevated blood calcium or high end of normal calcium.

Another example where the 1,25-D may be elevated is in *primary* hyperparathyroidism disease (pHPD). In about one third of pHPD cases, this hormone is elevated, and this condition causes bone loss and ultimately osteoporosis if undetected. pHPD also causes a low 25-D. The main differentiator is that in secondary hyperparathyroidism, caused by a vitamin D deficiency, the blood calcium is LOW, and in pHPD it is HIGH. However, vitamin D deficiency and pHPD can exist at the same time. This situation complicates the diagnosis and treatment requires a parathyroid expert.

The 1-25D test may also be elevated in conditions such as lymphoma or rheumatoid arthritis. Alternatively, a low level of 1,25-D can be associated with kidney disease or psoriasis. A further discussion of the 1,25-D test follows later in this chapter.

Which Test Is Better for Measuring Vitamin D Deficiencies?

Serum concentration of 25-D is the best indicator of vitamin D status and it has a half-life of 15 days. It reflects the vitamin D produced cutaneously as well as that obtained from food and supplements and has a fairly long circulating half-life of fifteen days. Circulating 1,25-D (active hormone) is not a good indicator of vitamin D status because it has a short half-life of fifteen hours, and serum concentrations are closely regulated.

Note: Half-life is the amount of time it takes for a substance to decrease by half, over a certain amount of time.

Interpreting Lab Results for the 25-D Test

When it comes to the 25-D test, it is good to have a basic understanding of what your test numbers mean, even if your report comes back in the normal range. Understanding your test numbers will help determine if vitamin D supplementation is necessary and, if so, how much you may need.

First, you should note which units of measurements are used to express the amount of vitamin D found in your blood. These units will usually be labeled ng/mL or nmol/L. The ng/mL measurement is the most common in the United States, and nmol/L is more common in other countries. Here's what those measurements mean:

NOTE:

Serum concentrations of 25-D are reported in both nanomoles per liter (nmol/L) and nanograms per milliliter (ng/mL).

ng/mL: nanograms per milliliter

nmol/L: nanomole per liter

1 nmol/L = 0.4 ng/mL

125 nmol/L is equal to 50 ng/mL

1 ng/mL is equal to 2.5 nmol/L

So, as an example, 50 ng/mL is equal to 125 nmol/L

Typically, with a 25-D test, you will see a number before the measurement of ng/mL or nmol/L, showing the amount of vitamin D in your bloodstream; for example, 15 ng/mL is the same as 37.5 nmol/L. Whether the numbers on your lab report can be considered "normal" or not is the subject of ongoing scientific debate.

The conventional wisdom for many years—which you will see listed in charts from governmental entities, from the Institute of Medicine (IOM) holds that a reading of only 20 ng/mL (or higher) is sufficient for bone and overall health. In my opinion, below 30 ng/mL is too low. While I do not agree with IOM, I am including the IOM recommendations for reference purposes. There are many variations regarding recommendations for the blood level of vitamin D. I am including the Endocrine Society and the Vitamin D Council.

25-Vitamin D Test Levels

Following are recommendations for the 25-D (Calcidiol) range guidelines from various organizations. I added my own preferred recommendations.

The following chart is adapted from the Vitamin D Council website.

The measurement for the numbers below is **ng/mL**

	Vitamin D Council	Endocrine Society	Dr. Lani's preferred recommendation	Institute of Medicine (IOM)	Testing Laboratories
Deficient	0–30	0–20	0–30	0–11	0–31
Insufficient	31–39	21–29	31–39	12–20	
Sufficient	40–80	30–100	40–50	>20	32–100
Toxic	>150		>150		

There are significant differences in the above recommendations regarding what is considered a vitamin D deficiency and sufficiency. My recommendations are most similar to the Vitamin D Council with the exception of the higher sufficient range that I do not recommend as safe or necessary.

Whether the lab results from your 25-D test are labeled "normal" or not, you need to keep these points in mind:

- A deficiency or insufficiency of vitamin D may not be obvious or produce overt symptoms.

  In winter months those who live below or above the 37-degree latitude do not make much, if any vitamin D from the sun and more vitamin D supplementation may be needed to maintain a healthy blood level.
- Long-term vitamin D deficiency or insufficiency can result in bone loss and potentially other health consequences as explained in chapter 5.
- It is impossible to determine an exact "optimal" or "ideal" vitamin D level for each individual. People who receive maximum sun exposure, such as lifeguards, exhibit naturally high blood levels of 25-D, roughly around 50 ng/mL, and some

studies have reported even higher serum levels in this select population.

■ Toxic levels of vitamin D in the charts above are very high. However, for some people a status over 50 ng/mL can be harmful if you have certain health conditions such as primary hyperparathyroidism, that you will learn about later in this chapter.

Some studies have shown that African Americans may need less vitamin D. This again is a debatable issue that has not been resolved. For African Americans 35-40ng/mL seems like a better range. The jury is still out.

Note: Recently, I had a 70 year old patient whose serum 25-D was 65 ng/mL and her serum calcium was 10.1 which is on the high end of the normal range. This level of serum calcium can point to primary hyperparathyroidism. Once she stopped vitamin D for 3 months her serum calcium returned to 9.5. She had been taking 5,000 IU daily. Now she is taking 3,000 IU. In this case her high vitamin D was resulting in a high end of normal serum calcium.

Vitamin D Test Results in a Nutshell

• Be sure to get the 25-D test—not the 1,25-D test—to determine your vitamin D status. The target for the 25-D test result is 40–50 ng/mL range (which translates to 100 to 125 nmol/L).

Dangerous Vitamin D Toxicity?

Vitamin D deficiencies are far more common than the extremely rare cases of vitamin D toxicity. Problems with prolonged high-end levels of vitamin D in the blood may pose risks too; some of these are known, and others may be revealed as more and more people supplement with vitamin D. This section explains some of the problems and precautions needed to avoid actual toxic levels.

We need to think about what a healthy blood level of vitamin D is, and that is around 40-50ng/mL. Remember that 1,000 IU typically increases the blood level by 10 points ng/mL. As an example, if someone naturally has a blood level of 30 ng/mL, then 1,000 to 2,000 IU is all they need to raise their blood level to 40–50 ng/mL. 5,000 could push their 25-D level to 70 or 80 ng/mL. I see no scientific evidence that over 50 ng/mL is better or heathier for the adult population at large.

When someone does exhibit problems from too much vitamin D, it is due to excess supplementation—not sun exposure—because, sun-induced D does not result in toxicity. At a certain point, after absorbing the sun's UVB rays and creating vitamin D, the human body shuts off production of D. The concern regarding vitamin D toxicity is centered on supplemental overdose, which is usually caused by an excessively high intake over a period of months.

Testing is the only way to make sure your blood level of vitamin D and calcium are balanced and at safe levels. Below you will see some of the indications of vitamin D toxicity. Hypercalcemia is primarily what causes the symptoms of vitamin D toxicity.

There have been cases of vitamin D toxicity that were due to incorrect dosing in a product. One spectacular example of this came from case of health advocate, Gary Null. He had his own supplement line and the lab made a big mistake—instead of 2,000 IU they put in 2,000,000 IU. Yes, you read that right, two million. After one-month Gary and six other people showed up at hospitals with severe kidney damage. You would think this level of overdose would kill someone, but it did not. However, it did result in severe hypercalcemia and kidney damage.

Vitamin D Toxicity Signs and Symptoms

The main consequence of vitamin D toxicity is a buildup of calcium in your blood (hypercalcemia), which can result in the symptoms listed below: Vitamin D toxicity can cause non-specific symptoms such as anorexia, weight loss, frequent urination, and heart arrhythmias.

When the 25-D test reports a level 150-200 ng/mL, for some, the toxicity symptoms below will be present. However, a 25-D level above 50ng/mL may result in health consequences for some and symptoms that may be more vague.

- hypercalcemia (elevated calcium in the blood)
- calcium deposits in the kidneys, lungs, blood vessels, heart, and other soft tissues
- kidney stones
  Hypercalciuria (increased urinary calcium excretion)
- irregular heartbeat
- weakness
- seizures
- nausea
- vomiting
- anorexia
- high blood pressure
- weight loss

The Vitamin D Council list has a slightly different set of symptoms that are relevant:

- hypercalcemia
- feeling sick or being sick
- having poor appetite or loss of appetite
- feeling very thirsty

- passing urine often
- having constipation or diarrhea
- abdominal pain
- muscle weakness or pain
- experiencing bone pain
- feeling confused
- feeling tired

NOTE: The number-one cause of hypercalcemia (elevated blood calcium) is due to primary hyperparathyroidism, which you will learn more about later in this chapter.

Now that you have a basic idea about what to expect from a test to check your level of 25-D, you may be ready to discover what particular dosage may be needed if you or a family member is deficient, or what you must do to maintain a healthy vitamin D status, plus a balance of other nutrients that work together with vitamin D.

But, before going on to the discussion of treatment/maintenance options (which you'll find in the next chapter), here is a quick look at the 1,25-D test.

Vitamin D 1,25-D Test: also called 1,25 Dihydroxy-vitamin D or Calcitriol

Calcitriol is the *active* form (hormone) of vitamin D. Remember that 25-D represents how much vitamin D we have on board, and it is not active until it goes through the kidneys, where it is converted into calcitriol. As mentioned earlier, the 1,25-D test has a short half-life and therefore is not tested to assess vitamin D status. However, I often order this test since I work with people who have been diagnosed with osteoporosis, and if it is high or low it helps with a diagnosis.

While most of this chapter focuses on the 25-D test, the 1,25-D test can help diagnose certain health conditions. Listed are some of the conditions associated with decreased 1,25-D as well as increased 1,25-D levels. As you can see from the chart below, an abnormal 1,25-D can be a very important diagnostic tool. Both low and elevated 1,25-D levels can be a sign of an underlying health condition.

1,25-D lab results

Low 1,25-D Level	Elevated 1,25-D Level
Vitamin D deficiency	Early vitamin D deficiency
Rickets	Primary hyperparathyroidism (pHPD)
Crohn's disease	Hypercalcemia (elevated blood calcium): One third of all cases are associated with pHPD. Also, with malignant lymphoma
Kidney disease	Rheumatoid arthritis
Type 1 vitamin D–resistant rickets	Sarcoidosis (vitamin D supplementation contraindicated)
Hypoparathyroidism	Women's menstrual cycle and pregnancy
Pseudohypoparathyroidism	Lymphoma
Psoriasis	Obesity
	Lyme disease
	Granulomatous diseases
	Tuberculosis
	Inflammatory bowel disease

Now that we have covered the vitamin D tests and results, we will focus on the importance of other tests that you may need to ensure your good health when considering vitamin D supplementation.

Understanding how the body regulates calcium in the blood is critical and that is what we'll cover next.

Calcium Regulation

Blood calcium is regulated by three major hormones: parathyroid hormone (PTH), calcitonin, and calcitriol (1,25-dihydroxyvitamin D [1,25$(OH)_2$D3]). Calcium regulation in the blood is tightly regulated. The acceptable range is not always healthy, as the high or low end of normal blood calcium could point to a significant health issue.

If the blood level of calcium is high (hypercalcemia) or low (hypocalcemia) this requires additional investigation. Low blood calcium is most commonly due to vitamin D deficiency. However, it also can be due to inadequate intake of calcium or malabsorption issues such as Crohn's disease or Celiac disease. Calcium absorption is strongly dependent on vitamin D levels. On the other hand, the most common cause of elevated calcium is primary hyperparathyroidism (pHPD). Primary hyperparathyroidism is a fairly common and often underdiagnosed condition. So, understanding how the parathyroid glands work is important.

There are four tiny (size of a grain of rice) parathyroid glands that are located behind the thyroid gland. One or more of these glands can enlarge (hypertrophy) or develop a small benign tumor (adenoma). Either condition increases bone loss over time because pHPD increases the release of its hormone parathormone. When elevated, this hormone releases calcium from the bones, and thus increases blood calcium. Because vitamin D increases calcium absorption, vitamin D supplementation can worsen the condition until the offending parathyroid gland or glands are removed. You can find more information regarding this condition online at parathyroid.com. In vitamin D deficiency, the parathormone also increases resulting in bone loss.

The following blood tests should be considered when vitamin D deficiency (Secondary hyperparathyroidism) is diagnosed. These are PTH-intact, serum calcium, magnesium RBC (red blood cell) and vitamin D (25-D). When osteoporosis is the diagnosis, I also order the 1,25-D test.

Normally, the parathyroid hormone helps regulate blood calcium levels; it is released whenever blood calcium levels are low. The parathyroid hormone increases blood calcium levels by stimulating osteoclasts, which break down bone to release calcium into the blood stream. If someone has chronically low calcium in their blood for any reason, the parathyroid glands will kick into gear, and more bone loss will occur. Think of the bone as a reservoir of nutrients, especially calcium, that the body will tap into if we do not get enough calcium. And yes, vitamin D deficiency can be the culprit if the calcium level is low, since vitamin D increases calcium absorption if the blood level is normal.

Typically, symptoms of elevated serum calcium, or hypercalcemia, are thought to be obviously symptomatic when serum calcium is above 12 mg/dL. In addition, you cannot feel bone loss or other developing diseases.

Normal Lab Ranges for PTH-Intact, Calcium, and Vitamin D:

I am including the normal lab test ranges that you will see on test results. However, a high or low end of normal can point to a serious problem. Depending on the lab, ranges may differ. While these "normal" ranges are on lab tests, many including myself do not consider the high and low ends necessarily normal. Following are the typical lab ranges for these tests.

- PTH-intact normal range: 10 to 55 pg/mL or 10 to 65 pg/mL
- Serum calcium: 8.5 to 10.3 (mg/dL)
- 25-D (25, hydroxyvitamin D): 30 to 100ng/mL

NOTE: Calcitonin Testing: Typically, the calcitonin test is only ordered if there is suspicion of thyroid cancer.

Important things to remember regarding test results:

- Elevated PTH and *low serum calcium* typically indicates vitamin D deficiency or deficient calcium absorption or intake.
- Elevated PTH and *elevated serum calcium* typically indicates primary hyperparathyroidism (pHPD).
- The most common cause of elevated blood calcium is due to pHPD.
- Sometimes the PTH test can be in the normal range, while calcium is elevated, or it is on the high end of normal—retest!
- The diagnosis for pHPD is primarily made following several serum calcium tests that are elevated, even when the pHPD test is in the normal range, assuming there is no other cause for elevated calcium.
- If serum calcium is low, and the 25-D is low, after 8 weeks of vitamin D3 therapy retest both nutrients.
- Generally, vitamin D supplementation is contraindicated if calcium is elevated until a diagnosis is clear by retesting. If your calcium is indeed high, or at the high end of normal, make sure you consult with a parathyroid expert to rule in or rule out pHPD.
- Also, pHPD can cause vitamin D deficiency and this is one reason, if you have questionable lab results, that you may need a specialist to sort it out.

There are other conditions that can result in elevated calcium (hypercalcemia) or low blood calcium. Aside from pHPD, conditions that can cause an elevated blood calcium includes cancer. Bottom line: don't ignore abnormal blood calcium test results.

My mentor, parathyroid expert Claude Arnaud, MD, once had me order twelve calcium tests on one patient as he suspected pHPD. Four were elevated and eight were in the "normal" range, but at the high end of normal. The patient did end up having parathyroid surgery to remove the gland and her blood calcium returned to normal. Besides vitamin D deficiency there are other causes of secondary hyperparathyroidism as listed below.

Causes of Secondary Hyperparathyroidism

There are several causes of secondary hyperparathyroidism, which are associated with poor absorption of calcium and vitamin D from the intestines or kidney disease. Some of the causes are listed below.

- Vitamin D deficiency over a prolonged period of time
- Kidney failure requiring dialysis
- Stomach or intestinal bypass surgery
- Celiac Disease
- Crohn's Disease

I was diagnosed with vitamin D deficiency 25 years ago. The lab results showed a low 25-D, an elevated 1,25-D and high end normal PTH-Intact, with a low end normal of serum calcium. This was corrected within 6 weeks following vitamin D3 supplementation. Because my calcium was *low* it was correctly diagnosed as secondary hyperparathyroidism.

Vitamin D Deficiency Masking Primary Hyperparathyroidism: 2004 Case Study

"Vitamin D deficiency and primary hyperparathyroidism (pHPD) are relatively common disorders. The coexistence of these conditions should be considered, as depletion of vitamin D may alter the clinical expression of autonomous parathyroid disease. We report details of a vitamin D deficient patient in whom replacement therapy led to the unmasking of occult pHPD."

In the case mentioned above, increasing this patient's vitamin D to a normal level resulted in an elevated serum calcium.

Keep in mind that pHPD is considered fairly common and results in an elevated serum calcium; it is suspected when serum calcium is on the high end of normal. Several calcium tests should be ordered to confirm an elevated serum calcium. In such cases, vitamin D is contraindicated, which is why it is important to check calcium before increasing vitamin D.

Besides the parathyroid concern, some people may show an increased serum calcium with increases of vitamin D at a 50+ ng/mL level. Clinically, I have seen elevated serum calcium with when the 25-D test was above 55ng/mL. These patients were taking vitamin D supplements and when they stopped vitamin D for two months their serum calcium returned to normal. In a discussion with surgeon and parathyroid expert Deva Boone, MD, she said that she too, has seen elevated serum calcium with a vitamin D blood level of 55ng/mL and higher.

After two to three months, it is also a good idea to recheck the 25-D along with calcium to make sure both are at a good level. I like to see calcium in mid-range or a bit lower—that would be 9.2 to 9.6 on average in adults over the age of 40, however, up to 9.9 can be normal for some of these people. That said, in pHPD the calcium can fluctuate from normal to elevated. This is why several tests may be needed to accurately diagnose.

The chart below is from the Norman Clinic (parathyroid.com) shows normal and abnormal serum calcium by age.

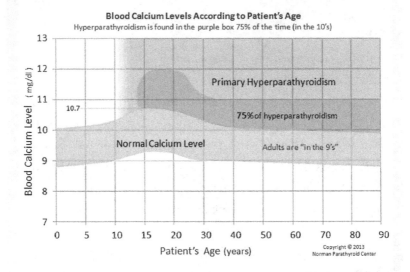

This chart shows abnormal and normal serum (blood) calcium levels by age. As you can see normal calcium does fluctuate with age. It also shows when serum calcium may indicate pHPD.

The following statement is from the parathyroid.com website:

"If you are over 35 years of age, and your blood calcium is *high* (over 10.1) you are almost certain to have primary hyperparathyroidism--a disease caused by a tumor. If your blood calcium is *high* and your vitamin D level is low, then you are almost guaranteed to have a parathyroid tumor (primary hyperparathyroidism)."

BOTTOM LINE: If you have an elevated blood calcium or high end of normal, make sure you work with a doctor who will evaluate your lab tests several times and include the 25-D test and the PTH-Intact tests.

Does Supplemental Vitamin D Cause Hypercalciuria (Elevated Urinary Output of Calcium)?

Studies have shown that high doses of vitamin D supplementation along with calcium supplementation can result in hypercalciuria and possibly kidney stones. This is another reason to make sure your vitamin D is at a good level, and that your calcium intake, from all sources, is not so high that it results in chronic, high urinary excretion of calcium. Some people consume too much calcium through a high dairy diet or supplementation and when the calcium is lowered, as well as the high dosing vitamin D, their 24-hour urine test can return to normal.

This points to how important it is to work with a well-informed health practitioner who will do proper testing that may include the twenty-four-hour urine test. For instance, all patients who have osteoporosis should have this test, as well as those who have a family history of kidney stones. Kidney stones are common in people who have pHPD.

Now that we have learned about testing for vitamin D and other important tests that may be needed before supplementing with vitamin D, we will now learn about the reliability of the vitamin D tests that are available from different laboratories.

Testing Methods (Assays/Testing Methods) for Vitamin D

There are many assays that labs use to measure vitamin D. The most reliable tests used today to test the 25-D are listed below. In 2017, the *Journal of Clinical Laboratory Analysis* evaluated the top two vitamin D testing methods. Concentrations measured by LC-MS/MS were higher than those measured by DiaSorin RIA, with a mean difference of 12.9 ng/mL. Following are the top two lab testing methods.

- DiaSorin Liaison (RIA) (immunochemiluminometric assay): Radioimmunoassay is considered the gold standard, because it was the one used in almost every major vitamin D study. Labcorp uses this method.
- LC-MS/MS: Liquid chromatography—on average, results are higher by 12.9 ng/mL. QuestDiagnostics uses this method.

Researcher Michael Holick recommends LC-MS/MS; many other researchers prefer the DiaSorin test. Mayo Clinic, Quest Labs, Esoterix, ZRT, and others use LC-MS/MS. Vitamin D experts are currently pressuring the lab industry to standardize all the labs.

Given the discrepancies, I decided to conduct my own small experiment. I went to LabCorp and QuestDiagnostics on the same morning to test for the 25-D and the ZRT blood spot test. Two friends also had their 25-D test done at both labs, but at different locations. The numbers represent ng/mL and the results were as follows:

Name	Quest Diagnostics	ZRT	LabCorp	Daily Vitamin D3 intake
Sandi	75.5/	70.7		4,000 IU D3 past 3 months
Mari-Claire	63.0	62.1		5,000 IU for one year
Lani	48.0	49.0	47.7	4,000 IU ~ 6 months
1,25-D				
Lani	66.0		65.4	

While this was a tiny sample of 3 different people at different locations I was impressed with the close results. What do I glean from these tests? I recommend not testing at other labs that do not use these two testing methods. The blood spot test from ZRT was reliable, although I was the only one that did this test. Rarely is a lab test of any kind 100% reliable. I recommend going to either lab and if you retest, use the same lab as there are some differences.

In this chapter, we have learned that opinions regarding vitamin D testing, and what the blood level of the vitamin D test (25-D) should be, varies significantly, depending on the source. The Institute of Medicine has one recommendation, while some highly respected researchers feel that the IOM recommendations are far too low. My opinion is most similar to the alternative recommendations mentioned earlier. I've also discussed how we should not take vitamin D supplementation lightly, as vitamin D in its active form is a powerful hormone. It is now up to you to determine how much supplementation you and your family may require, in addition to the UVB rays from sun exposure in your area. The best way to get an idea about your vitamin D level is to test your levels.

In the next chapter you will learn about various options for increasing vitamin D if you are deficient, sources of vitamin D, and how D supplements are manufactured.

Key Points from Chapter 6 — Vitamin D Testing and Associated Tests

- The 25-hydroxyVitaminD (25-D) is the correct vitamin D test to check your serum level
- The target for vitamin D serum level is 45ng/mL

■ Vitamin D is contraindicated if serum calcium is on the high end of normal or elevated

■ Primary Hyperparathyroidism is the most common reason for high serum calcium

■ Caution is advised regarding how much vitamin D to take

■ The range that most people need to supplement is between 1,000-4,000 IU daily, depending on UVB ray exposure

■ Magnesium is important for proper functioning of the parathyroid gland

Chapter 7

Vitamin D Recommendations

In the previous chapter, we learned about vitamin D testing, and the different opinions regarding how much vitamin D you and your family actually need. For decades, the U.S. government's official policy stated that most adults under age seventy needed only 200 to 400 IU (international units) to maintain an adequate intake (AI) of vitamin D daily. Currently, the National Institutes of Medicine (IOM) at the National Institutes of Health has increased that dosage to 400 to 800 IU of vitamin D daily. The latest recommended dietary allowance (RDA) for vitamin D was officially set in 2016 and in 2019 the recommendations are still the same.

Yet, if you ask many of the leading vitamin D researchers, they would tell you that the RDA is far too low, and that most healthy adults require approximately 2,000 to 4,000 IUs of vitamin D on a daily basis, from a *combination* of sun and oral ingestion, to maintain a healthy blood level of vitamin D, especially during winter months. The healthy target level that I recommend is 45ng/mL.

If you are deemed to be vitamin D deficient by a health-care provider, you might be prescribed as little as 800 IU, or as much as 10,000 IU daily, for a number of weeks, or permanently. Or you might be prescribed a single weekly dose of 50,000 IUs, of either vitamin D3 or D2. Vitamin D2 (ergocalciferol), as will be discussed later in the chapter, is not recommended as the best source for vitamin D. Needless to say, these vastly different recommendations are confusing.

And, regarding high dosing all of the sudden—what's the hurry? If we have had a vitamin D deficiency for a while, or even years, our bodies have acclimated to it. Given that research in this area is scant at best, in my opinion, it is better to raise the level more slowly over a two to three-month period. This is because vitamin D will significantly increase absorption of calcium and raise the blood calcium level. For some, this rapid increase may be a problem and potentially harmful. In my opinion starting with 1,000 IU to 2,000 IU for the first 4 weeks is more reasonable and increasing the dose as needed to achieve the target goal of 45 ng/mL.

Vitamin D Dosage on Supplement Labels

Both International Units (IU) and micrograms (µg) are used as measurements that you will see on supplement labels. In the United States, vitamin D is typically measured by International Units (IU). Countries that use the metric system use micrograms as the measurement that you will see on their labeling system. 1,000 IU of vitamin D is equivalent to 25 micrograms.

Keep in mind that there are small studies that have shown that the body can produce a significant amount of vitamin D in one day. Research in a controlled laboratory setting has shown that a young adult, who is exposed to UVB rays, with a UVB lamp, can produce 10,000 IU in one day, with 85 percent of the body exposed to UVB rays. This study gained popularity in the alternative health world, and many doctors thought that if the body can produce 10,000 IU daily then that amount is safe and preferred to take as a daily dose.

The 50,000 IU prescription that medical doctors often recommend as a weekly dose originated because it was easier to give it to patients in nursing homes. I am cautious when recommendations far exceed what the body would naturally produce from UVB exposure or intake from dietary sources. As of this writing, there is not enough evidence to convince me that long-term high doses, or even short-term oral high doses, are safe for the majority of people who take them. Later in this chapter, I offer my views regarding what I consider to be safer dosage recommendations.

You can find references on the Internet regarding doctors who are currently treating patients for conditions such as multiple sclerosis, tuberculosis, and other diseases with very high doses of vitamin D, sometimes in the hundreds of thousands of IUs. For the most part, these doctors are not practicing in the United States. I mention this with extreme caution regarding treating diseases and conditions with excessively high doses of vitamin D, as we simply do not know what the long-term effects might be, or whether or not it is an effective treatment option. The research is ongoing, however, so more will be revealed in years to come.

With this wide range of recommendations, it's no wonder that people are confused and that a number of myths and misconceptions have arisen about the amount of vitamin D each person requires.

Fortunately, it is possible to work your way through these various recommendations to determine the appropriate amount of vitamin D that you may need. This chapter is designed to help with that process, so you can find out whether or not supplementation is right for you and, if so, how to tailor a program that will work for the individual needs of your family.

Before looking at your individual needs, it is helpful to know a little about how vitamin D recommendations are set for the general population, and that is the focus of the next two sections.

Is Taking Vitamin D supplementation the same as getting Vitamin D from the sun?

No, it is not. Remember from earlier chapters that other substances are produced at the same time we produce vitamin D3 when we expose our skin to the sun's UVB rays. We are just beginning to understand the importance of these other substances and how they may benefit our body, as well as potentially work with vitamin D3. In fact, we have found at least one of them in the blood as well as the adrenal glands.

Your Daily D

It is of utmost importance to understand that vitamins A, D, E, and K are fat-soluble vitamins. So, if you take any of these nutrients as a supplement, you will not absorb them unless you take them with food that contains fat. I have had many people tell me that their vitamin D blood level is low, despite the fact that they take a supplement, only to find out that they were taking vitamin D in-between meals or before going to bed.

When looking at a bottle of vitamins or a food label, you are probably accustomed to seeing a nutritional value listing for the contents, and you may be familiar with the term *recommended dietary allowance* (RDA). Two other common terms are *adequate intake* (AI) and *upper limit* (UL).

- RDA—Recommended Dietary Allowance: The RDA represents the average daily intake that is *sufficient* to meet the nutritional requirements of nearly all healthy individuals (97 to 98 percent) in each age and gender group.
- UL—Tolerable Upper Intake Level: The UL identifies the maximum daily intake unlikely to cause adverse health effects.

■ AI—Adequate Intake: The AI level is established when evidence is insufficient to develop an RDA. The AI is set at a level assumed to ensure only nutritional adequacy. Presently an RDA has been established for vitamin D; however, you will see AI mentioned in many articles or research papers prior to the new RDA recommendations.

Some of the past and current controversies that have swirled around vitamin D concern the UL safety limit and the RDA. The Institute of Medicine recommends lower levels of both, which many vitamin D researchers dispute, as you will see below.

The following section discusses these intake recommendations—and the differences between what I refer to as the "official recommendations" and alternatives to those recommendations.

Vitamin D Recommendations

To give you a baseline understanding about vitamin D recommendations, let's begin with a look at the recommendations from the Institute of Medicine (IOM). Below is a list that shows the 2019 RDA values, and the second table shows the tolerable upper intake level (UL). Many vitamin D researchers, and others like me, think that the RDA is too low.

The other important question is whether or not it is wise to recommend vitamin D first, without testing the blood level of vitamin D. How much vitamin D is safe, and what are the contraindications for vitamin D? You will find the answers to these questions later in this chapter. For now, we will look at official and alternative recommendations for vitamin D that are based on minimal sun exposure. Following are the official recommendations from IOM.

IU stands for international units, and is the measurement most often used for vitamin D in the United States. Also, micrograms, or μg, are the metric measurement for vitamin D commonly used in Europe. IUs convert to micrograms (μg) at a ratio of 40 to 1, that is, 40 IU = 1 μg. First we will look at the RDA recommendations from the IOM and then the alternative RDA recommendations.

Official RDA for Vitamin D

- 0 to 12 months*: 400–600 IU for males and females
- 1 to 70 years old: 600 IU (this includes pregnancy and lactation)
- Over 70 years old: 800 IU

*0 to 12 months Adequate Intake (AI)—the RDA has not been established

Official Vitamin D Tolerable Upper Intake Level

- 0 to 6 months: 1,000 IU
- 9 to 18 years: 4,000 IU
- 19+ years: 4,000 IU

Vitamin D Intake—Alternative Views

I have been working on this book on and off for over ten years. During this time, I have attended vitamin D conferences, interviewed researchers, attended presentations, and read countless research papers and books on the topic. Many viewpoints and critiques have shaped my views regarding vitamin D. There are varying recommendations by the IOM; Endocrine Society; Michael Holick, MD; many others. There are two charts. The first chart is from the Endocrine Society and then Michael Holick.

The Endocrine Society recommends the following for vitamin D supplementation:

Note: AI is used not RDA because they are not a government agency.

Endocrine Society
2018 Recommendations for Adequate Intake and Safe Upper Limit

Age groups and special groups	AI	Safe Upper Limit
0 to 6 months	400 IU	1,000 IU
6 mo. to 1 year	400 IU	1,500 IU
1 to 3 years old	600 IU	2,500 IU
4 to 8 years old	600 IU	3,000 IU
Older than 8 years	600 IU	4,000 IU
0 to 1 year old	400 IU	4,000 IU
1 + years old	600 IU	4,000 IU
19 to 50 years old	600 IU	4,000 IU
50 to 70 years old	600 IU	4,000 IU
Over age 70	800 IU	4,000 IU
Obese individuals	2 to 3 times more than above	No recommendations
Pregnant and nursing women	600 IU	No recommendations

Michael Holick, MD: Dr. Holick's current recommendations for vitamin D are listed below, to show a comparison to the government's recommendations. Holick's UL is much higher (10,000 or adults) and unless there is a clinical reason the the vitamin D test is low, I do not agree that up to 10,000 is safe or preferable. I agree, for the most part, with his AI level.

Below are Dr. Holick's recommendations for vitamin D intake, from all sources, which may include some vitamin D from the sun, nutritional sources, and supplements. I list his chart as a comparison to the IOM recommendations. Note: AI is used here instead of the RDA which is the official recommendation.

Michael Holick MD
2018 Recommendations for Adequate Intake and Safe Upper Limit

Age groups and special groups	AI	Safe Upper Limit
0 to 1 years old	400 to 1,000 IU 10 mcg to 25 mcg	2,000 IU* 50 mcg
1 to 12 years old	1,000 to 2,000 IU 25 mcg to 50 mcg	4,000 IU* 125 mcg
13+ years old through adulthood	1,500 to 2,000 IU 38 mcg to 50 mcg	10,000 IU 250 mcg
Pregnant and nursing women	1,500 to 2,000 IU	10,000 IU

Egad! Now what? As you can see, all three recommendations are different. First, we need to know how much vitamin D the adult human body utilizes. I am not aware of studies that definitively quantify this. However, in an interview with vitamin D researcher Robert Heaney, he stated that, in his opinion, that amount is about 4,000 IU each day, from *all sources*, for most adults. The above recommendations are assuming a small amount of sunlight.

Tolerable Upper Intake Limit UL and Safe Upper Limit (SL) Concerns

When most people see the UL or SL they will assume that the amount listed is *safe*. The UL listed by IOM is 4,000 IU and Michael Holick's is as high as 10,000 IU. Keep in mind that 40-50 ng/mL, is the target range that I recommend as safe for most people and 3,000 to 10,000 IUs can put them in a much higher range. Remember, it depends on how much vitamin D you are getting from the sun. I would stick to the AI recommendations and I strongly recommend vitamin D testing with calcium for the best results. Keep in mind that vitamin D, in its active form (1,25-D), is a powerful hormone.

Some examples of those who may need higher vitamin D doses include those who have conditions such as fat malabsorption, kidney problems, obesity and other conditions. However, someone without such conditions may also show unexpected low 25-D levels. If this is the case, make sure vitamin D is consumed with a fatty meal.

Many people may take high doses of vitamin D without balancing other important nutrients such as calcium, magnesium, vitamin K2, and others. These nutrients support both heart and bone health and, in my opinion, are critical when supplementing with vitamin D. Studies have shown that low and elevated vitamin D can result in atherosclerosis.

Vitamin D Upper Tolerable Intake Level (UTL)

Note that the IOM refers to the UTL and the alternative recommendations use the term Safe Upper Limit (USL). The only reason some people may need higher doses such as 5,000 to 10,000 IUs every day, is if they have some condition that prevents them from achieving the target of 45ng/mL. My opinion regarding the USL is partly based on the concern about high serum calcium levels, that are not known unless it is tested. Taking as much as 10,000 IU could result in health consequences, and for some, raise their blood level over 100 ng/mL. It is speculation that a blood level above 50 ng/mL is needed and healthy for most people. For me the jury is still out.

Below is a list of my recommendations and considerations before taking vitamin D supplementation.

Dr. Simpson's Vitamin D Recommendations and Tips:

After reviewing varying opinions from existing research papers, from respected cancer groups and doctors, and from the IOM, my recommendations are as follows:

- Before vitamin D is added as a supplement, it is prudent to test your D level when possible, and I strongly recommend that blood calcium level is tested too.

- Vitamin D is fat soluble and must be ingested with a fatty meal.

- Once you know your calcium level is okay, then begin to replenish vitamin D, if your D level is low. Most doctors prescribe a very high dose of vitamin D with the idea to increase vitamin D as fast as possible. There are no long-term studies that indicate this is safe.

- The vitamin D test target range that is safe for most people is 40 ng/mL to 50 ng/mL.

- Keep in mind that when you supplement with D3 it takes 6 to 8 weeks to increase your blood level, so it is best to retest after 8 weeks. If you supplement with D2 (not recommended), it will take up to three months to achieve the same level.

- For people who live in northern latitudes, or who for one reason or another are not getting much vitamin D through sun exposure, 1,000 to 2,000 IU is a good amount to start with, especially during winter months when vitamin D production is low or non-existent. As an example, 1,000 IU will be enough for someone who tested at 35 ng/mL. In this case, the added 1,000 IU daily should increase the 25-D to 45ng/mL. If for some reason this level is not achieved, then adding another 1,000 IU should be sufficient.

  Test serum calcium to make sure it is mid-range normal—remember that even a high-end range normal of calcium needs to be investigated.

- Some doctors recommend as much as 10,000 IU daily for their patients. This much vitamin D would put most people at a higher blood level of the 25-D test at around 100 ng/mL, and I do not recommend such high doses, unless clinically necessary to achieve the target range. Some people do need higher levels, due to digestive problems or some other issue related to absorption of this fat-soluble vitamin.

- Vitamin D does not act alone. It is important to maintain a healthy diet and lifestyle, and not regard vitamin D supplementation as a panacea.

- Take vitamin D earlier in the day rather than at nighttime. Some people's experience and some small studies show that there could be a relationship between sleeping difficulties and late ingestion of vitamin D. The hypothesis is that vitamin D might decrease melatonin production if taken late at night (see Chapter 13 for more information on melatonin).

NOTE: If an individual's vitamin D blood level is naturally high due to sun production, that is fine, but in my experience it is rare in Northern California. Recently, one of my patients boasted being outside every day surfing—midday, in the summer, in Southern California with no sun protection. He is in his fifties, and his blood level measured 50 ng/mL.

Vitamin D Does Not Act Alone—Vitamin K2 to the Rescue.

Vitamin D needs helpers and supporters known as co-factors in order to function optimally in our bodies. Magnesium and vitamin K2 are two of the most important nutrients to include if you are not getting enough from foods. It is difficult to get enough of either of these nutrients from the diet. While there are many other nutrients that impact vitamin D, we will focus these two nutrients.

Vitamin K2: As mentioned above, vitamin D ensures that your blood level of calcium is high enough to meet your body's demands.

However, vitamin D does not fully control where the calcium in your body ends up. That's where vitamin K2 steps in.

Vitamin K2 regulates calcium in your body in at least two ways:

- **Promotes calcification of bone:** Vitamin K2 activates osteocalcin, a protein that promotes the accumulation of calcium in your bones and teeth.

- **Reduces calcification of soft tissues:** Vitamin K2 prevents calcium from accumulating in soft tissues, such as the kidneys and blood vessels.

How much vitamin K2 do we need?

Author Kate Rheaume-Bleue, BSc, ND, Vitamin K2 and the Calcium Paradox, **How a Little Known Vitamin Could Save Your Life** recommends the following:

There are two sources of K2—MK4 (menaquinone) and MK7 (menaquinone). MK7 is the preferred source. A maintenance dose of 100 mcg of vitamin K2 (MK7) is fine for most people. However, a higher intake of 180 mcg. for people with conditions such as osteoporosis or atherosclerosis is a better target. It is hard to get this much from foods alone unless you eat Natto (fermented soy). If you would like more detailed information about K2, I suggest reading Dr. Rheaume-Bleue's book.

Magnesium:

Inadequate magnesium is common, in fact, muscle cramps that can be due to a lack of calcium could also be caused by insufficient magnesium. Here are some points to consider about magnesium.

- High doses of vitamin D can deplete magnesium.
- Previous research has suggested that **magnesium** may reduce the risk of **vitamin D** deficiency.

- It is critical to balance calcium with magnesium, with at least a 2:1 ratio (calcium to magnesium).
- The serum levels of parathyroid hormone and magnesium depend on each other in a complex manner.
- Magnesium may help vitamin D activate vitamin D into Calcitriol—more research is needed.

How much magnesium do we need?

It is critical to balance magnesium with calcium in at least a 2:1 ratio (calcium to magnesium). Calcium intake, from all sources should be between 900-1,200 mg daily unless there is a clinical reason to add more. There are many forms of magnesium—one of the best is magnesium glycinate that is more absorbable than other forms. Magnesium in other forms, such as oxide or citrate are not as well absorbed. Magnesium can result in loose stools for some, especially those that are not well absorbed. This could be a welcome relief for those who suffer from constipation.

Can you take too much magnesium? Yes, and less is known about how much is too much. What is known is that magnesium is tightly regulated in the body so, to be safe I would use the 2:1 ratio mentioned above.

Summary: One of vitamin D's main functions is to ensure adequate levels of calcium in your blood. Vitamin K2 promotes calcium accumulation in your bones, while reducing its accumulation in soft tissues such as blood vessels.

Does Supplemental Vitamin D Cause Hypercalciuria (elevated urinary output of Calcium)?

Studies have shown that vitamin D supplementation along with high calcium intake from the diet or calcium supplementation can result in hypercalciuria and possibly kidney stones. This points to how important it is to work with a well-informed health practitioner who will do proper testing that may include the 24-hour urine test if indicated. For instance, all patients who have osteoporosis should have this test, as well as those who have a family history of kidney stones. If calcium is elevated in urine, and especially in the blood, primary hyperparathyroidism could also be the culprit.

Concerns regarding increasing vitamin D too fast: Many people consume a significant amount of calcium from dairy products and supplementation. Let's say they have been deficient in vitamin D for years and, all of a sudden, the vitamin D level goes from 15 ng/mL to 50 ng/mL. Vitamin D will increase calcium and phosphorus absorption by 50 percent, so they will be absorbed twice as much as before and this may not be a good thing for some people.

However, many people also consume diets very high in calcium from dairy products. In these cases, the increase of calcium absorption can be high. So why is high calcium so bad? The body must eliminate excess calcium. Most excess goes out through the kidneys, and chronically high excretion of calcium through the kidneys may result in kidney stones, and some excess calcium may also precipitate into body tissues. Many people suffer from chronic constipation because they absorb too much calcium. There are other reasons such as balancing calcium with magnesium and being hydrated that will be discussed in chapter 8.

Let's add one more confounding issue—many people eat a diet that is high in sugar and processed carbohydrates, drink alcohol, and some smoke cigarettes and consume too much meat and animal products. This type of diet and lifestyle increases inflammation in the body, and calcium tends to accumulate in areas of inflammation! This is why it is important to work with a health-care practitioner who will look at your entire health picture before simply adding vitamin D supplementation.

Vitamin D—Get What You Need

You now have a great deal of information to answer the question posed at the beginning of this chapter: How much vitamin D do you really need? You know about the recommendations for vitamin D intake from conventional and cutting-edge researchers, as well as my assessments of those recommendations. Now it's up to you to take this information and put it to use. I encourage you to find out what your body needs by getting tested for your current vitamin D level. With those results in hand, you can find that place of balanced optimal nutrition through the multiple sources of vitamin D available— sunlight, food, and supplements. Exactly how and in what proportion you use these sources depends on your personal needs and your lifestyle. In the next chapter you will learn about how to increase your vitamin D level to a safe level if you are low in this critical nutrient.

Key Points from Chapter 7 — Vitamin D Recommendations

■ Vitamins A, D, E, and K are fat-soluble vitamins

■ RDA—Recommended Dietary Allowance is set very low for vitamin D

■ Opinions vary greatly regarding how much vitamin D we need

■ A vitamin D blood level of 45 ng/mL is a healthy target for your vitamin D status

- 1,000 IU of vitamin D should increase your blood level 10 ng/mL

- Taking high doses of vitamin D is contraindicated for some people

- If the serum calcium is elevated, vitamin D is contraindicated

- Vitamin D does not act alone. Calcium, magnesium and vitamin K2 are important

Chapter 8

Treating Vitamin D Deficiencies

Suppose your lab tests come back showing that you have a deficiency for vitamin D. In this section, you'll learn what you and your health-care provider can do to treat that problem and, it is hoped, to set up a program for maintaining a healthy level of vitamin D.

Before giving you details about treatment and supplementation, however, here are a few points I need to stress.

- First, if you are lacking this important vitamin, your short-term and long-term health can be significantly impacted. So, you will need to work on shoring up your levels of D through diet, sensible sunbathing (See Chapter 11), and supplements when it is appropriate.
- And the second point is: We still don't know everything! So, before considering your treatment options, please heed this caution. Right now, a groundswell of excitement surrounds the role vitamin D plays in a wide array of disease processes and medical conditions. Overall, I'm very happy about this increased awareness and acceptance of what we in the nutritional health community have been asserting for a long time. That said, you and your doctor need to be careful about supplementing with vitamin D, as I have previously discussed in Chapter 7. For some people, vitamin D supplementation is contraindicated.

As we learned in the previous chapter, vitamin D does have an upper limit of safety. The Office of Dietary Supplements sets their Tolerable Upper Intake Level for vitamin D at 4,000 IU, and some alternative recommendations are as high as at 10,000 IU and higher. Unfortunately, when the average person reads these recommendations, they may think that 4,000 or 10,000 is safe and healthier, and that simply is not the case.

When medical doctors treat a patient, who is vitamin D deficient, they often prescribe 50,000 IU weekly or 10,000 IU/day for 6–8 weeks or indefinitely. The prescription is often D2 (ergocalciferol)—which is not the best choice, because vitamin D3 is superior to D2. Another treatment some doctors have used is a once-a-year dose of 200,000 IU—that's right, 200,000. Needless to say, some people who received this dose did not fare well.

My preferred program for treating vitamin D deficiency is using D3 supplements that can be purchased at a health food store and that can be taken orally. I also have preferences when it comes to the sources used for vitamin D. Doses ranging from 1,000 IU to 10,000 IU can be purchased from health food stores or alternative doctors. I strongly favor a regimen where supplemental vitamin D is taken in smaller, daily amounts rather than a prescription of 50,000 IU in one weekly dose. That is because I think it is best, whenever possible, to follow what nature intended for our bodies to produce naturally and the body never produces 50,000 IU of vitamin D in one day.

When someone has been deficient for a long time, is it a good idea to flood their body with high doses immediately? This is what almost all doctors of any persuasion recommend. However, I have given this a lot of thought, and I think it is more prudent to start with lower amounts of 1,000 to 2,000 IU for a number of weeks, while nutrition status is assessed by a nutrition specialist to make sure important nutrients (see below in nutrition section) are balanced. I have had two patients who reported ending up in the emergency room with severe chest pains following taking 50,000 IU. Maybe it was not related to the chest pain, but it did make me think through the common practice, and I am more comfortable starting slowly. Slowly, because their body has not had a healthy level for some time, and as mentioned in earlier chapters, calcium and phosphorus absorption will be significantly increased once 25-D (calcidiol) converts to hormone D (calcitriol) within two months. In addition, as mentioned in Chapter 7, other nutrients should be balanced with vitamin D supplementation.

For certain individuals who are unable to absorb vitamin D due to surgical removal of the intestines, kidney disease, or some other reason, an injectable form of vitamin D may be prescribed. Also, people in this situation might consider another option, which is the use of a UVB-producing sun lamp (see Chapter X for more details) or transdermal or sublingual vitamin D3.

Studies regarding vitamin D supplementation for transdermal (skin application) have shown that vitamin D is absorbed through the skin. Exactly how much it will raise the blood level is not clear. Sublingual (under the tongue) has also been shown to increase the blood level in patients with Crohn's disease. Both of these options should be considered when oral dosing is not effective.

Formula for Vitamin D Supplementation

A healthy person who takes 1,000 IU of vitamin D3 should show an increased blood level of about 10 ng/mL (25 nmol/L). Keep in mind that you must take vitamin D with a fatty meal. Vegans typically do not ingest as much fat as carnivores. So, if you are on a low-fat diet for any reason, make sure you take in fat when supplementing. Sometimes I will have an avocado or a lot of olive oil added to my meals to make sure that I absorb vitamin D as well as the other fat-soluble vitamins A, E and K.

How long does it take to convert 25-D to the active hormone 1,25-D? The answer is six to eight weeks. I have tested well over 1,000 people in the past twenty years, and I find that this result is typically true, if the patient does not have a problem with absorption. D2 takes up to three months to convert to the active hormone.

For example, if your vitamin D level is 20 ng/mL and you want to raise it to my recommended blood level of 40-50 ng/mL, then 2,000 IU should get you there or very close. Your blood level does not need to be perfect, as our blood level changes day to day, depending on UVB exposure and the vitamin D we obtain from food, which is not significant.

Is there a formula regarding how much vitamin D we need based on height and weight? The Vitamin D Council adds that the size of a person matters regarding how much vitamin D we need to take. So, larger people may need more to achieve similar results, though there is no exact formula regarding height and weight. The body mass index does make a difference, that is, how much fat versus muscle on an individual basis. Also, males may need more than females to achive the target serum level of vitamin D.

Which Is Better, Vitamin D3 or Vitamin D2?

When considering vitamin D supplementation, it is important to consider this question: Is the D3 (cholecalciferol) form of vitamin D better than D2 (ergocalciferol)? The answer to this question is that D3 is hands down the best. Canadian researcher Rhinehold Vieth, PhD, puts it this way. D2 is less stable. He concludes that D3 is the best choice, because D3 it is exactly what the body produces naturally when the skin is exposed to UVB rays. Vitamin D3 could be more than three times as effective as vitamin D2 in raising the blood level of 25-D and maintaining those levels for a longer period of time. Now that we know that D3 is preferable to D2, let's look at how both vitamins are manufactured.

Manufacturing of D3 (Cholecalciferol)

The commercial production of vitamin D3 relies primarily on animal sources and one plant source:

- Lanolin: Lamb's wool gives us lanolin, which is the primary source used today to produce vitamin D3 supplementation. After a purification process and crystallization, it is converted into 7-dehydrocholesterol that is the specific form of cholesterol required to produce vitamin D3. Vitamin D is also obtained via an organic solvent extraction of the animal skins of cows, pigs, or sheep followed by an extensive purification process.

   Once vitamin D, from any source, is chemically pure, it is impossible to determine the original animal source (fish, sheep lanolin, pig skin, cow skin, etc.). It is then subjected to UVB radiation that transforms the substance to D3.

- Fish oil: D3 from fish oil is extracted and made into supplements. D3 from fish must also be purified.

- Lichen: This source of D3 is made from lichen and it is the *only* vegan (non-animal) source of D3. Lichen (which are small, algae-like plants) produce and accumulate D3 and other nutrients as they grow. The lichen is gathered and washed at the site where it is found, then sent away for processing. I was unable to determine the exact extraction methods used to produce D3. This source of D3 is more expensive than animal-sourced vitamin D.

Ergocalciferol Vitamin D2

This form of vitamin D is derived from fungus or yeast. It is typically produced synthetically from radiating (UVB rays) a compound (ergosterol) from the mold ergot. mushrooms, especially Shiitake mushrooms that are exposed to UVB rays are popular among vegetarians. Non-dairy milk substitutes, including soymilk, almond, and rice milk are fortified with 100 IU D2 per 8 ounces. (Cow's milk is fortified with 100 IU D3 per 8 ounces.)

Can You Mix Vitamin D and Your Medications?

Besides recognizing how the different forms of vitamin D can affect your body as explained in the section above, it is also important to understand what happens to this vitamin when it interacts with medications. Certain medications can interfere with the absorption of vitamin D, can decrease vitamin D concentration, or otherwise might interfere with conversion to the hormone vitamin D (1,25-D). Surprisingly, some of these are over-the-counter medications.

Below you will see a list of the prescription drugs that are known to interfere with vitamin D absorption. If you are taking any of the medications on this list, check with your physician, pharmacist, or other health-care provider before taking supplemental vitamin D. Unfortunately, many people in the medical field may not be up-to-date on the latest information about vitamin D and medication concerns. As the patient, then, you will need to do some homework on your own and be sure to ask about your health-care provider's familiarity with the issues surrounding vitamin D supplementation.

Following is a list of medications provided by the National Institutes of Health regarding medication interactions with vitamin D.

Steroids: Corticosteroid medications such as prednisone, often prescribed to reduce inflammation, can reduce calcium absorption and impair vitamin D metabolism. These effects can further contribute to the loss of bone and the development of osteoporosis associated with their long-term use.

Osteoporosis Medications: Teriparatide (Forteo) is a medication that builds new bone and at the same time removes old bone. Forteo decreases 25-D (calcidiol) and increases the active hormone (calcitriol) 1,25-D. This reaction is similar to what is seen in primary hyperparathyroidism and secondary hyperparathyroidism. **Tymlos** (Abaloparatide) is a newer medication that is similar to Forteo. Both medications are parathyroid analogues. Vitamin D and serum calcium need to be monitored when taking either medicaition.

Other Medications: Both the weight-loss drug orlistat (brand names Xenical and Alli) and the cholesterol-lowering drug cholestyramine (brand names Questran, LoCholest, and Prevalite) can reduce the absorption of vitamin D and other fat-soluble vitamins. Both phenobarbital and phenytoin (brand name Dilantin), used to prevent and control epileptic seizures, increase the hepatic metabolism of vitamin D to inactive compounds and reduce calcium absorption. It is always a good idea to check what medications interfere with vitamin D and to clearly know the side effects of the drug. Following are additional medications that can interfere with vitamin D.

- anticonvulsants
- barbiturates
- cholestyramine
- cimetidine (Tagamet)
- colestipol
- diuretics
- heparin
- isoniazid (INH) and rifampin
- ketoconazole
- mineral oil laxatives
- orlistat
- phenytoin (Dilantin)

- primidone (Mysoline)
- valproic acid (Depakene)
- phenobarbital
- calcium channel-blockers
- thiazide diuretics

Animals Need Vitamin D Too

We see our indoor pets seeking the "sun spot" on the floor to take a nap. However, windows block UVB rays, so unless they can get some unfiltered sunlight when UVB rays are present, they will not produce vitamin D. Furry mammals, including our cats and dogs, obtain the bulk of their vitamin D from licking their fur, and birds get it from preening their feathers.

Unlike humans and reptiles, cats and dogs do not make vitamin D in their skin. When UVB rays strike an animal's fur, oils in the fur are activated to produce vitamin D.

Animals, like humans, can suffer deficiencies of vitamin D. Unfortunately for indoor pets, lying by a window that filters out almost all UVB rays will not produce vitamin D. Animals need to be in direct, unfiltered sunlight when UVB rays are strongest at midday.

Dr. Michael Holick has been on a mission to educate zoos and pet owners regarding the need for UVB lamps for some of their indoor reptile residents. If iguanas, for instance, are kept indoors without sunlight, their bones soften, and they develop rickets. And resident tortoises display shells that look damaged with crevasses rather than a smooth surface, a sign of vitamin D deficiency. A simple UVB lamp can provide the needed natural vitamin D–producing rays. It can be purchased at many pet stores and easily attaches to a reptile's cage.

Contraindications for Vitamin D Supplementation

Correcting a vitamin D deficiency may worsen some conditions such as autoimmune disorders. Vitamin D, in its most potent form, is a powerful hormone and an antioxidant that increases immune system function. So, those who have autoimmune conditions, such as lupus and other conditions listed below, should be monitored carefully and closely if supplementation is suggested.

There are conditions where vitamin D supplementation is contraindicated, such as:

- hypercalcemia (elevated blood calcium)
- primary hyperparathyroidism with high serum (blood) calcium levels
- sarcoidosis
- rheumatoid arthritis (RA) (While studies have implicated vitamin D deficiency as a trigger in developing RA, once RA is established, 1,25-D may be elevated.)
- hypervitaminosis D: excessive vitamin D in blood
- tuberculosis: may become hypercalcemic when given increased vitamin D doses
- lymphoma: may become hypercalcemic when given increased vitamin D doses
- multiple myeloma
- abnormal sensitivity to the toxic effects of vitamin D
- history of kidney stone
- kidney disease with reduction in kidney function
- high amount of phosphate in the blood
- high amount of calcium in the blood
- arteriosclerosis with occlusion of the arteries

Vitamin D and Your Diet

Up to this point, we have discussed using supplements to remedy deficiencies or to maintain a healthy level of vitamin D. But what about getting vitamin D from your diet?

In the United States, vitamin D is added to milk and other common foods found on supermarket shelves, including breakfast cereals; however, the amounts are very small. Milk is fortified with vitamin D3. Each quart contains 400 IU, which breaks down to 100 IU per glass of milk. In terms of vitamin D intake, milk *should* contain fat—as vitamin D is a fat-soluble vitamin. (Other dairy products, including yogurt, cheese, and butter, are not fortified with vitamin D.) Children who do not drink milk, and who are constantly protected from the sun or don't spend much time outdoors, are especially at risk for vitamin D deficiency.

> **Note of caution!** Fetuses and breastfed infants are particularly at risk for vitamin D deficiencies unless the mother is taking supplementation.

Check labels on products, food items, and supplements that you consume regularly to see what your average daily intake might be from all sources. Many non-dairy products fortify their product with D2 (ergocalciferol). Because D2 is produced from plants, it is usually acceptable to vegetarians. I have stated my preference for supplementing with D3 (see section on "D2 or D3—Which Is Better?"), and I do not have a problem with the D2 in non-dairy milk products. But these products contain only a small amount of D2, and when you are estimating total dietary vitamin D intake, remember that D2 is half as potent as D3.

The chart below from the National Institutes of Health shows that it is difficult to obtain significant levels of vitamin D from food sources alone, unless you are opting for cod liver oil, which I do not recommend in high doses. (See the cod liver oil debate below.)

Food Sources of Vitamin D3

Vitamin D3 is superior to D2. The chart below is only for D3. The best supplemental source for vegans and vegetairans is D3 sourced from lichen. D2 is not recommended as the primary source for vitamin D.

Food	International Units (IU) per serving
Cod liver oil, 1 tablespoon	1,360
Salmon, cooked, 3½ ounces	360
Mackerel, cooked, 3½ ounces	345
Tuna fish, canned in oil, 3 ounces	200
Sardines, canned in oil, drained, 1¾ ounces	250
Milk, vitamin D fortified, 1 cup	98
Egg, 1 whole (vitamin D is found in egg yolk)	20
Liver, beef, cooked, 3½ ounces	15
Cheese, Swiss, 1 ounce	12

The Cod Liver Oil Debate

Relatively little vitamin D is found naturally in the foods we eat, and diet alone will not provide enough to maintain a healthy store. One exception is cod liver oil, which is rich in vitamin D. One tablespoon of cod liver oil can contain as much as 1,300 IU of vitamin D, and the amount of vitamin A can vary significantly. One concern about cod liver oil is it's high vitamin A content. Remember, like vitamin D, vitamin A is a fat-soluble vitamin that accumulates over time in fat tissue. Claude Arnaud, MD, one of the world's top bone experts, points out that vitamin A stimulates bone cells (osteoclasts) to "chew up" bone. Thus, he advises against high vitamin A intake through diet and supplementation. Therefore, if you have low bone mass or if you are at risk for osteoporosis, a high intake of vitamin A is contraindicated, and that includes cod liver oil.

Our bodies have a great way to make sure we do not become toxic with vitamin A: the body makes it as it needs it. The liver converts provitamin A substances—some beta-carotenes and carotenoids—to produce a fat-soluble form of vitamin A (retinol). Not everyone converts these substances to vitamin A, and some do need supplementation. If you are concerned or know you have liver disease you can have your vitamin A (retinol) checked with your next blood test from your doctor.

Beta-carotene is an important antioxidant that the body converts to vitamin A, and it is found in a variety of fruits and vegetables.

Provitamin A substances are naturally occurring pigments found in plants and are largely responsible for the vibrant colors of some fruits and vegetables. Beta-carotene, for example, is responsible for giving carrots their orange color.

Another concern regarding cod liver oil is how it is processed—how do we get that oil out of the livers of cod fish? The extraction method is a long process that includes solvents. Also, many cod liver oils don't have the original vitamin A (retinol) in the product and instead add synthetic vitamin A (palmitate) back into the "purified oil." For this and other reasons, I do not recommend taking cod liver oil.

Pregnant Women, Developing Fetuses, Infants, and New Mothers

Fetuses require vitamin D for tissue development, including the skeletal structure, nervous system, and brain. Studies have shown that pregnant women are as frequently deficient as the rest of the population. Vitamin D is critical for fetal development. Therefore, I strongly recommend vitamin D testing for women who are considering pregnancy and want to ensure the very best outcome for bearing a healthy infant. For pregnant women, vitamin D testing should be included as a new standard for prenatal care. I say this with full awareness that the cost of testing can be a financial burden, but the benefits of providing the best in utero environment will ultimately prove to be cost effective. Healthy fetal development of bones, organs, and brain is worth the cost, if you can possibly manage it. Pregnant and lactating women may need to supplement with 4,000 IU to 6,000 IU/daily to achieve and maintain the target vitamin D level of 45 ng/mL.

Infants, too, require vitamin D. Studies have shown that human breast milk does not contain enough vitamin D to support the robust needs of an infant. Breast milk can range from 5 IU to 140 IU of vitamin D per liter of breast milk. Infants need a minimum of 400 IU each day. Pregnant women and mothers should maintain a healthy vitamin D blood level of 40 to 50 ng/mL. Some supplement companies offer vitamin D drops that are a great option for infants or anyone who cannot swallow a pill.

Another factor is this: if a pregnant or breastfeeding woman is deficient in vitamin D she, too, will suffer the consequences of deficiency if she is not meeting the demands of the developing fetus or nursing infant that requires significant amounts of calcium. As we learned earlier, vitamin D increases calcium absorption by as much as 50 percent and maybe even more during pregnancy.

Pregnancy and Lactation Osteoporosis (PLO)

PLO is often diagnosed following one or more fractures that occur during the birth process or after birth. Little is known about this condition. I suspect some of these women may have had low bone density prior to birth and low vitamin D or calcium intake during pregnancy and lactation. This could push their bones over the edge and result in fractures. One of my patients, at the age of 35, endured eight spinal fractures, that were related to PLO.

New mothers, too, may fair better with the demands of motherhood with optimal vitamin D stores. Although postpartum depression has several potential causes, vitamin D is certainly on the list of possible therapies to consider, particularly because of the known link between depression and vitamin D deficiency.

American Academy of Pediatrics Increases Vitamin D Recommendations

In 2008, the AAP issued a report recommending intakes of vitamin D that exceed those of the Food and Nutrition Board (FNB). The AAP recommendations are based on evidence from more recent clinical trials and the history of safe use of 400 IU/day of vitamin D in pediatric and adolescent populations. AAP recommends the following:

- 400 IU/day for exclusively and partially breastfed infants. Start a supplement of vitamin D shortly after birth and continue until they are weaned.
- Similarly, all non-breastfed infants ingesting less than 1,000 mL/day of vitamin D-fortified formula or milk should receive a vitamin D supplement of 400 IU/day.

- Older children and adolescents who do not obtain 400 IU/
  day through vitamin D-fortified milk and foods should take a
  400 IU vitamin D supplement daily.

All milk sold in the United States provides up to 100 IU of vitamin D3 per 8 ounces. The majority of vitamin D supplements are 400 IU. Multivitamins usually provide 400 IU per serving.

How Much Vitamin D do Infants and Children Need?

In Chapter 7 we reviewed different opinions regarding vitamin D intake recommendations for infants and children from 1 to 12 years old. I am most comfortable with 1,000 IU to 2,000 IU adequate intake recommendation that Dr. Michael Holick recommends.

Adolescents

Michael Holick, PhD, who has studied adolescents in Maine and elsewhere, estimates that as many as 30 percent of adolescents nationwide may be affected by a chronic vitamin D deficiency. He estimates percentages among Blacks are probably even higher. "It's really an unrecognized epidemic," Holick said. It's no wonder that many adolescents are vitamin D deficient. Electronic gaming, web surfing, TV/DVD viewing—all indoor activities—have supplanted recreation such as sports, which required kids to be outside in their spare time. That and shunning vitamin D-fortified milk in favor of soda results in adolescents having significantly less opportunity to take in even the minimum level of vitamin D for good health. So here, too, is a population identified as, "at-risk" for vitamin D deficiency who would benefit from a routine daily supplement.

In this chapter, we have learned that vitamin D supplementation should not be taken lightly. Deficiency in this vital nutrient is not healthy and may lead to many illnesses. We live in a world unlike our ancestors, who were outside much of the day in the sun. Fortunately, with the knowledge that we have today, we can make sure that we have a healthy vitamin D level for ourselves and our family, though we must be aware of the risks. In the next chapter, we will learn about what can happen if we overindulge in sun exposure, and the risks of skin cancer.

Key Points from Chapter 8 — Treating Vitamin D Deficiencies

- Take vitamin D supplements with a fatty meal

- A vegan form of vitamin D3 is available. It is made from lichen

- Vitamin D2 (ergocalciferol) is derived from fungus or yeast.

- Vitamin D2 is not the best form of vitamin D and is not recommended

- Cow's milk is fortified with 100 IU per 8-ounce glass of milk

- Some medications interfere with vitamin D

- Vitamin D increases calcium and phosphorus absorption

- Some osteoporosis medications decrease vitamin D stores in the body

- Fetuses and breastfed infants are particularly at risk for vitamin D deficiencies, unless the mother is taking supplementation.

Chapter 9

When the Sun Is Too Much— Skin Cancer Risks

Hailed for millennia as a life-giving deity, the sun now bears one title that is far from noble: carcinogenic. The *Fourteenth Report on Carcinogens* from the Department of Health and Human Services provides a list of known and probable carcinogenic substances that includes ultraviolet radiation exposure as a carcinogen. They mention UVA, UVB, and sun lamps and sunbeds—anything that emits ultraviolet radiation. The sun is included in the list, along with tobacco smoking and other carcinogens, because of the link between excessive solar and other sources of UVR radiation exposure and skin cancer.

Besides reducing one of the most powerful forces in the universe to a carcinogen, the report does not include a number of important factors. For one, it does not address the sun dosage that is required to be labeled as harmful. So, while the list rightfully underscores the cancer-causing potential of sunburns and excessive sun exposure—which is a point I agree with—it does not offer any guidelines or research findings about sensible sun exposure. Nor does it address the potential benefits of sun exposure, such as the sun's role in producing vitamin D in our bodies. And producing vitamin D—as we now know from the latest research—can inhibit some cancers (such as colon, prostate, and breast), which may be more life threatening than skin cancer.

Despite these shortcomings, some government advisors, dermatologists' associations, and sunscreen manufacturers maintain that you should stay out of the sun as much as possible, especially

between the hours of 10:00 a.m. and 2:00 p.m., and obtain vitamin D from supplements or food. And some overzealous doctors
have gone so far as to claim that even sensible sun exposure should
be avoided because it could prove carcinogenic.

Instead of buying into such an extreme point of view and/or
being paralyzed with fear about contracting skin cancer, it is much
healthier to develop a mindful, sensible relationship with the sun.
And that means this: just as you have learned about how the sun
can help you—by building vitamin D stores—so, too, it is important
to understand the ways in which the sun can harm you, whether
through excessive sun exposure that results in sunburn or through
excessive lifetime exposure that may trigger skin cancer. Then you
can assess your personal risks and make informed decisions about
how best to protect yourself and your family.

One of the first problems you will encounter in trying to understand the sun's carcinogenic potential is the fact that skin cancer can
run the gamut from annoying or troublesome to disfiguring and even
deadly. Because the most common types of skin cancer are rarely
fatal, and more than 90 percent are easily removable in the early
stages, some people ignore the warning signs and fail to take reasonable precautions. And though the overwhelming majority of skin
cancers are not likely to kill you, one form of the disease, melanoma,
is a serious condition that can metastasize and lead to death. It's
important, therefore, for you to know how the various types of skin
cancer develop, what you can do to avoid them, and how to get
early treatment before they cause local damage or metastasize.

In this chapter, then, we will begin with an explanation of how
excessive exposure to ultraviolet (UV) radiation can potentially lead
to pre-cancers and skin cancer. You will also learn some reasons for
the apparent rise in skin cancer cases over the past several decades,
the most common risk factors for the disease, and the distinctions

among the various forms of it. Further, you will read about the need for and the limitations of, conducting skin self-examinations, as well as the vital importance of protecting your eyes. The misuse of sunscreens and indoor tanning facilities is also linked to a rise in skin cancer, and those issues are discussed in Chapter 11. Subsequent chapters will focus on skin cancer prevention and treatments, while this one will give you the basic concepts and vocabulary you need to understand this condition.

Skin Cancer and the Sun

First, let's take a look at the mechanism that turns the ultraviolet rays of the sun into a force that can damage skin cells and set up the conditions for cancer. The threat of skin cancer is far less frightening when you become familiar with the basic processes underlying this condition.

In terms of how cancer operates, one way to understand the general consensus view among scientists today is to think of the disease as "cells gone wild" or a cellular "failure to communicate." Normally, an orderly process governs the division and growth of cells in your body as they go about the business of repairing or replacing damage at the cellular level. The skin is an active site for this type of activity, as new skin cells push older ones up to the surface of the body where they die and, eventually, slough off. This process is run by specific genes in your DNA, which tell the cells when to start and when to stop the division process. If that DNA is damaged, the stop-and-go signals to the cells can get scrambled. So, they may "go wild" and start dividing out of control, setting the stage for cancer.

This process can be likened to the children's game of "gossip" or "rumors," in which one person whispers something to the person in the next chair, and that person repeats what he or she heard to the next person, and so on around the circle. By the time the message gets to the last person, it is usually so mixed up that everyone has a good laugh.

Unfortunately, this process is not so funny when it takes place in the cells of your body and the clear instructions that should pass from cell to cell get mangled; the result can be cancerous, as the cells start growing out of control. *So, how does this process apply to skin cancer?* Read on.

How Sunburn Damages Skin Cells

If you've ever experienced sunburn, you don't need anyone to tell you what it is. But in technical terms, the National Institutes of Health (NIH) officially defines sunburn in this way: "A sunburn is reddening of the skin that occurs after you are exposed to the sun or other ultraviolet light." The NIH report also describes the cause of this condition in this way: "Sunburn results when the amount of exposure to the sun or other ultraviolet light source exceeds the ability of the body's protective pigment, melanin, to protect the skin. Sunburn in a very light-skinned person may occur in less than fifteen minutes of midday sun exposure, while a dark-skinned person may tolerate the same exposure for hours." All of that said, however, it is important to remember that dark-skinned people also suffer sunburns.

The definitions and distinctions from the NIH are useful for scientists and researchers. It is far easier, however, to simply remember this: Sunburn is essentially an inflammation of the skin. In addition to the reddening and inflammation that you can see on the surface of your body, sunburns also cause damage you cannot see because when ultraviolet radiation—or UV rays—penetrates the skin, it damages the DNA in your skin cells. With any type of inflammation, the body's repair system goes into action to "clean up" the problem. But if the body's "repair crew" misses any of the damaged cells, they can eventually evolve into cancer. Instead of being sloughed off through the normal regeneration of your skin, the "broken" cells left behind by the "repair crew" linger and mutate—which is why a sunburn at age sixteen could produce skin cancers decades later.

The most common of skin cancers, which account for about 95 percent of all skin cancers, are basal cell and squamous cell carcinomas. Both of these non-melanoma cancers (keratinocyte carcinomas) can develop from sunburned skin as well as from excessive long-term sun exposure or cumulative damage; however, squamous cell carcinoma is more associated with excessive cumulative damage. You'll see details on these forms of skin cancer in the sections that follow, but the main thing to know about them is that they rarely spread beyond a localized area when they are caught early. The more serious form of skin cancer—melanoma—also can develop following DNA damage. In regard to sun exposure, it is most associated with sunburns, though cumulative, long-term damage also plays a role. Interestingly some melanomas occur on areas of the body that are not exposed to the sun.

According to the Skin Cancer Foundation, "The sun exposure pattern believed to result in melanoma is that of brief, intense exposure, like a blistering sunburn, rather than years of tanning."

UVB rays burn the skin, and UVA rays tan the skin. However, both UVB and UVA rays can trigger cellular changes—DNA damage—that can result in skin cancer.

This diagram illustrates how a sunburn can evolve to skin cancer years later from damaged cells.

Sunburn
⇓
Body mops ups damaged cells.
⇓
Some damaged cells with damaged DNA remain.
⇓
Years later, damaged cells can evolve into cancerous or pre-cancer lesions.

What's Behind the Rise in Skin Cancer?

Now that you have a general understanding of how skin cancer develops, it's important to get some perspective on why you hear so much in the media about the dangers of this condition. The general consensus is that all forms of skin cancer have steadily increased over the past fifty or more years. Below you will see some of the basic facts reported by the Skin Cancer Foundation, followed by a list of factors that may be contributing to its rise.

Skin cancer by the numbers:

- Skin cancer is the most common form of cancer.
- More than three million cases are diagnosed in the United States each year.

However:

- Less than one percent of all cancer deaths are from skin cancer.
- Skin cancer is cured 85 to 99 percent of the time.

Note these facts too:

- Non-melanoma has a high cure rate when detected early.
- The five-year survival rate for people whose melanoma is detected and treated before it spreads to the lymph nodes is 99 percent.
- Melanoma accounts for 75 percent of skin cancer deaths.

Nevertheless:

- 40 to 50 percent of Americans who live to age 65 will have skin cancer at least once.
- Skin cancers of any kind can be disfiguring, especially in sensitive areas of the face: nose, ears, lips, and eyelids.

Dermatologists often contend that skin cancer rates are increasing because people are staying out in the sun too much while also not protecting themselves properly with sunscreen. While this is certainly part of the equation for some, it is also important to point out that before the advent of sunscreen products, most people had much more sun exposure, especially on the head and arms.

Undeniably, cumulative, excessive sun exposure and blistering sunburns are clearly linked to skin cancer, but how can these facts alone account for the substantial increased rate of skin cancer? Some possible explanations follow.

Longevity: People Are Living Longer, Thus More Skin Cancers Will Develop

Baby boomers are growing older. The millions of baby boomers, who were growing up in the United States after World War II, often tanned and burned their skin in pursuit of a "healthy glow." Today, that population group is getting older, and the damage done to their bodies decades ago may be showing up as skin cancer today. Another reason for the increase in skin cancer diagnosis is that more people are seeing dermatologists today and getting diagnosed, which is a good thing.

False Sense of Security from Sunscreen Use

People think sunscreens protect their skin and, therefore, they need not worry about the sun. Believing their skin is protected, they assume they can expose their skin safely, and often for extended periods of time during midday. This is a false assumption propagated by the sunscreen industry. Not all skin damage is visible.

Lack of UVA Protection in Sunscreens

UVA rays have a longer wavelength than UVB rays. UVA rays penetrate deeply into the skin, and most sunscreen chemicals do not offer good protection from this ray. Unfortunately, early sunscreen chemicals did not offer any UVA protection. Since UVA rays do not burn the skin, like UVB rays, people are often unaware that these UVA rays are damaging their skin.

Sunscreen chemicals and other ingredients in sun products: There are many photo-biological studies that show the harmful effects of some sunscreen chemicals on living tissue. Some researchers hypothesize that a percentage of skin cancers may be the direct result of free radical damage caused by these chemicals. This question is explored further in Chapter X. It is not good sun sense to allow your skin to be exposed to the sun for multiple hours regardless of what type of sunscreen you're using. This practice will result in skin damage.

Vacation travel: Our ancestors did not have the ability to hop on a plane and land thousands of miles away within hours. Now it is common for large numbers of people to travel far from their home latitudes and subject their skin to sudden bursts of intensive sun exposure on vacation, which perfectly positions them for sunburns and, potentially, skin cancer.

Indoor tanning: UV radiation at tanning salons also causes damage that may trigger skin cancer. The increased use of tanning beds has been linked to a rise in melanoma among young people and, some doctors suggest, melanoma of the eye. The UVA rays tan the skin, and in sunbeds these rays can be more than ten times the strength of sun-produced UVA rays.

Poor diets: The *Standard American Diet* (SAD) tends to include excessive intake of junk foods that are high in processed carbohydrates with sugar and poor-quality fats. The SAD diet is likely another factor in the rise of skin cancer. The skin, like the heart and bones, requires an array of nutrients to be healthy. Vegetables and fruits are loaded with skin nutrients, and antioxidants, such as vitamins A and C, as well as vitamin D, are needed for good skin health. These nutrients protect the skin and some studies suggest that they even prevent some sun damage.

All of the above factors explain why skin cancer rates seem to rise every year. But how do these considerations apply to you personally? In the next section, you will get an overview of the main factors that can put you, individually, at risk for developing skin cancer.

Are You at Risk for Skin Cancer?

Clearly, people with lighter skin are more susceptible to sunburns and are at greatest risk for skin cancer. However, people of color also contract skin cancer, and they need to practice good sun sense too. In fact, people with dark skin are often not diagnosed as skin cancers can be more difficult to diagnose. As you read about risk factors below, keep in mind that this list covers general categories and you will need to carefully assess your own personal status in consultation with your health-care provider. You'll also find more information on detecting skin cancer warning signs later in this chapter.

Risk Factors for Developing Skin Cancer and Pre-Cancer Lesions

- Light, sun-sensitive skin, particularly among those with light-colored hair (red or blond) and light-colored eyes.
- Sunburns: Blistering sunburns result in the most skin damage. Sunburns at any time in life increase the risk of skin cancer. Sunburns before the age of eighteen double the risk of skin cancer later in life.
- Age: Since most sun-related skin cancers develop slowly, the risk of being diagnosed goes up as a person ages.

- Excessive, cumulative sun exposure, especially as seen in out-door workers (such as fishermen, farmers, or construction workers), surfers, skiers, etc.
- Frequent use of tanning salons: Here the risk may be due to the high-intensity bursts of UVA radiation, which can be up to ten times stronger than the UVA rays emitted by the sun.
- Personal and/or family history: Anyone who has had skin cancer runs the risk of developing it again, as does someone who has a first-degree relative (parent or sibling) who has had the disease.
- Moles: Having multiple moles and atypical moles increases risk.
- Cigarette smoking, excessive alcohol consumption, and drug use.
- Weakened immune system, such as people with HIV/AIDS or leukemia.
- Conditions that weaken the skin or blood circulation, such as diabetes.
- Poor nutrition, particularly diets low in antioxidants, high in unhealthy fats, and marked by processed carbohydrates and sugar.
- Sunny or high elevations: UVA and UVB rays are more intense at high altitudes or in sun-intense areas.
- Occupational or environmental hazard exposures, especially to coal tar, pitch, creosote, arsenic compounds, or radium.
- The medical procedure to treat certain cancers with radiation increases the risk of skin cancer in the exposed area.
- Medications and herbs: Certain medications can make your skin more sensitive to sun exposure. Some of these medications include antibiotics, certain cholesterol-lowering medications, high blood pressure and diabetes medications, and

non-steroidal anti-inflammatory drugs such as ibuprofen (Advil, Motrin, others). Particular herbs, such as feverfew and St. John's wort, also make the skin more susceptible to sunburn. Ask your pharmacist if the medications you take will make your skin more sensitive to sun exposure.

When you hear about skin cancer risks, remember that all risk factors are not created equal. Someone with a family history of melanoma (specifically, an individual with a parent or sibling who's had the disease) will probably have a higher risk than a person whose distant cousin once had skin cancer. Also, as you can see from the above risk factors, your personal habits and environmental exposures play a significant role. The next section will explain pre-cancers and the differences among the major forms of skin cancer so you can become better versed in this subject and, thus, more able to accurately evaluate your risks. Following you will learn about pre-cancer lesions (Actinic Keratosis).

Nutrition for Skin Health

One of the most important things you can do to avoid skin cancer is to eat a diet that supports healthy skin. As it turns out, this is the same diet that is good for our bones and heart. Many years ago, I had a moment that changed my relationship with food forever. The very first time I walked into a health food store in 1971, I immediately spotted a book whose title was, *You Are What You Eat* by Adele Davis. At that time, I thought, "If this is true, I am in trouble." My diet was not good, and I was addicted to sugar and processed carbohydrates. What is a healthy diet? There are many opinions regarding eating a healthy diet, but I think author Michael Pollan sums it up pretty well with his trademark statement: "Eat food. Not too much. Mostly plants."

In essence this means we should eat a diet that is high in fiber and colorful foods that will boost the intake of antioxidants, eat more vegetables than fruit, and eliminate, as much as possible, processed carbohydrates and sugar. In addition, research shows that antioxidants reduce the severity of a sunburn as well as provide some protection against skin cancer. Of course, as with everything else we discover through research, a little common sense is called for. A few alternative doctors have claimed that eating a diet high in antioxidants will actually stop sunburns. That is simply not the case, and everyone needs to practice safe sun sense and protect the skin—no matter what quantity of fruits and vegetables are consumed. In the next chapter, you will learn more about nutrition and skin health.

It is a known fact that a healthy diet does reduce skin lesions and pre-cancers.

Actinic Keratosis (Solar Keratosis):

Actinic keratosis (AK), also known as "pre-cancer," can resemble a dry patch of skin or an active lesion that is red and tender. Sometimes lesions can start as an itchy bump that looks like a small pimple. An estimated 10 percent of active lesions, which are redder in color and more tender or itchy than the rest, will progress to squamous cell carcinoma. Most AK is not active, and, as noted, can simply appear as a dry patch of skin.

Actinic Keratosis Risk Factors:

- It is more common in light-skinned people who lack the melanin found in dark skin to protect them.
- 40 to 60 percent of squamous cell carcinoma begins in untreated AK lesions.

- If you have AK, it indicates that you have sustained sun damage, and any kind of skin cancer can develop, not only squamous cell carcinoma.
- Cell damage caused by cumulative sun exposure can cause DNA damage that eventually may result in AK development.
- It is most common in people who have had considerable sun exposure: outdoor workers, surfers, and other outside sporting activities.
- AK is most common closest to the equator or Southern Hemisphere where the sun is more intense. Light-skinned people living in these areas are at higher risk.
- People whose immune systems are suppressed as a result of chemotherapy, AIDS, organ transplantation, or other immune-suppressing conditions are also at higher risk.

Actinic Keratosis Characteristics:

Mostly, these dry, scaly areas are annoying. However, if they span a large area on the face, or if they appear on the lips, nose, or ears, they can be much more problematic. If you find a suspicious area, see a dermatologist. Most are easily treated, but characteristics include:

- common appearance on the face, lips, ears, scalp, neck, backs of the hands and forearms, shoulders, and back.
- measurement of one-eighth to one-fourth inch in size and may appear in small clusters.
- may appear and disappear in early stages.
- a lesion that is flat or raised with a dry and rough, scaly, or crust-like appearance.
- often these lesions are felt first, before seeing them, due to the roughness.

- itchiness.
- ill-defined borders.
- variety of color: dark or light, tan, pink, or a combination.
- the appearance can resemble a small pimple or scab.
- patches may itch occasionally and bleed.

Actinic keratosis, as noted above, can be a pre-cursor to squamous cell carcinoma. Now we will examine the types of skin cancer lesions.

Types of Skin Cancer

There are two main types—melanoma and non-melanoma, with basal and squamous cell carcinomas being included in the non-melanoma group. We will focus on the distinctions among basal cell carcinoma, squamous cell carcinoma, and melanoma. As you read this section, keep in mind that all types of skin cancer can develop anywhere on the body. In fact, sometimes skin cancers that arise in non–sun exposed areas can be the most aggressive. While skin cancer can be divided into several categories and subcategories, three major types exist:

- basal cell carcinoma
- squamous cell carcinoma
- melanoma

Below, you'll see basic overviews of these various forms of skin cancer:

Basal Cell Carcinoma (BCC)

Basal cell carcinoma (BCC) is the most common skin cancer, comprising of 70 to 80 percent of all skin cancers. This cancer arises in the outer layer of the skin, called the epidermis. In the

United States, the occurrence is approximately 150 to 300 per 100,000 people, while in Australia, it is approximately 1,000 per 100,000. Men are affected more often than women, due to outdoor work; however, women who work outdoors are also at greater risk. Even though BCC is a form of skin cancer, some refer to it as the "friendly cancer" because it rarely metastasizes. However, it certainly is not friendly if it develops on sensitive body sites such as the nose, lips, or even the genital area. More often than not, these superficial cancers are easily removed and will not recur, but that is no reason to ignore the importance of keeping your skin protected appropriately, as fully discussed in the chapter on sensible sun exposure (see Chapter 11).

My Personal Experience with Over Twenty BCC

One of the reasons I wrote this book is because of my own experience with skin cancer. As of this writing, I have had over twenty BCC and one SCC in-situ. As I shared in the introduction, I lived in the sun as a child and every year suffered multiple severe, blistering sunburns. My first skin cancer showed up around the age of forty and I did not have it checked out for years, despite the fact that it bled occasionally. Fortunately, it was on my back and easily removed, requiring only ten stitches. Today, almost thirty years later, I find my skin cancers before my dermatologist, through self-examination (covered later in this chapter). I now practice sun sense (as discussed in Chapter 2) religiously, as I am well aware that I am at high risk for all forms of skin cancer due to my personal history of severe sunburns, chronic unprotected sun exposure, and multiple skin cancer diagnoses.

Basal Cell Carcinoma in a Nutshell

- BCC is the most common form of skin cancer and there are many subtypes that you will learn about in the next chapter. The most common are superficial; however, some can be deep and destructive.
- BCC is commonly seen on the face, ears, neck, scalp, shoulders, and back. While this is a so-called *friendly* cancer, remember that BCC can become a costly, and possibly disfiguring, problem if it is discovered on the face and on areas such as the ears, eyelid, lips, or nose.
- Sunburns any time in life, and especially early in life, can set the stage for BCC to develop years later. Also, excessive lifetime exposure is a risk factor.
- Mostly associated with UVB rays (the ones that cause sunburn).
- Most instances of BCC are superficial and rarely metastasize. (This means they do not travel to other parts of the body.)
- BCC can cause extensive local damage if left untreated.
- This form of cancer can also arise on areas of the body that are not sun exposed.
- This form usually grows slowly and may take years to be noticed.
- It can be removed or treated topically.
- It is most common in light-skinned people with light eye color.
- In some cases, contact with arsenic, exposure to radiation, and complications from burns, scars, and vaccinations can all be contributing factors.

Will Tattoos Increase the Risk of Skin Cancer?

The inks used in tattoos have thus far not been shown to increase the risk of skin cancer recurrence. People who have had skin cancer are always at higher risk of developing future skin cancers, but tattoos do not increase that risk. However, tattoos may make it difficult to notice skin changes, which may prevent early detection and diagnosis in some cases.

Squamous Cell Carcinoma (SCC)

Squamous cell carcinoma (SCC) is the second most common skin cancer, comprising 15 percent of all skin cancers. SCC forms in squamous cells (flat cells that form the surface of the skin). It is primarily attributed to cumulative lifetime sun exposure, but sunburns can also set the stage for the development of SCC. Frequent use of indoor tanning also multiplies the risk of SCC; people who use tanning beds are 2.5 times more likely to develop SCC than those who don't. Skin injuries are another important source. The cancer can arise in burns, scars, ulcers, long-standing sores, and sites previously exposed to X-rays or certain chemicals (such as arsenic and petroleum by-product).

Squamous Cell Carcinoma in a Nutshell

- Many SCC arise in areas that were previously diagnosed as actinic keratosis (pre-cancer lesions).
- Approximately 3 percent of squamous cell carcinomas will metastasize if left untreated.
- SCC is common to areas of the body that have endured significant cumulative sun exposure, such as the face, nose, shoulders, etc.
- It also can arise on areas of the body that are not sun exposed.
- SCC is usually superficial but can be invasive.
- It is associated with the deep-penetrating UVA rays as well as UVB rays.
- Some cases of SCC are related to human papilloma virus.

■ Actinic cheilitis is an aggressive form of SCC that appears on the lips and can evolve into squamous cell carcinoma. An estimated one-fifth of this type can metastasize if not treated.

NOTE: Oral cancer is frequently a form of squamous cell carcinoma. In addition to tobacco and alcohol, human papilloma virus (HPV) is associated with a proportion of the head and neck cancers. This is why dentists should check the tongue and surrounding tissues. If you have a sore in the mouth that is not healing, have it checked out.

Melanoma

In the 1930s, the lifetime risk of an American developing invasive malignant melanoma was 1 in 1,500. That risk as of 2014 is 1 in 36 for men and 1 in 58 for women, according to the American Cancer Society website. In a report published by Darrell Rigel, MD, in the journal *Seminars in Cutaneous Medicine and Surgery*, he pointed out that melanoma is one of the few remaining cancers with increasing U.S. incidence and that the mortality rate from this disease has risen about 2 percent annually since 1960.

The American Cancer Society notes that increases in the incident rates for melanoma "have been most pronounced in young white women and in older white men." People with darker skin, however, are not immune from melanoma. In fact, because of the prevailing myth that people of color are not susceptible to melanoma, they may be diagnosed only after it has advanced to a late stage, when it is harder to treat and more likely to prove fatal. (For more on this issue, see the section below entitled "**Marley's Melanoma: An Example of Skin Cancer in Dark Skin**," which points out, among other things, that even though he had dark skin, the famous reggae musician, Bob Marley, succumbed to melanoma.)

All forms of melanoma are serious; however, some are much more aggressive than others, and virtually all forms are treatable if caught early. Melanoma has been linked to severe sunburns at any age, but particularly to those occurring before the age of eighteen. There is growing evidence that short bursts of intense UVA rays used in tanning salons may also increase the risk of developing melanoma. More than just the sun is at work in the expression of melanoma, however, as you can see in the list of risk factors for this condition further below.

Medical Paradox: Melanoma and the Navy

Starting with the hypothesis that exposure to the sun's UV rays causes the most serious form of skin cancer, melanoma, it would seem logical to conclude that people working outdoors would have a higher incidence of this disease than those whose occupations keep them indoors. A famous study of Navy personnel, however, found the opposite to be the case. Personnel who spent most of their time indoors at their desks actually had a higher rate of melanoma than sailors who worked outdoors. The study, *Occupational Sunlight Exposure and Melanoma in the U.S. Navy*, reported that: "Compared with the U.S. civilian population, personnel in indoor occupations had a higher age-adjusted incidence rate of melanoma. Incidence rates of melanoma were higher on the trunk than on the more commonly sunlight-exposed head and arms." Interestingly, because of the location of the melanomas—and the fact that people who alternated their time between indoors and outdoors had the lowest rates of melanoma—the study suggested that vitamin D production might have played a protective role in suppressing the growth of malignant melanoma cells. As the report (published in the

Archives of Environmental Health) stated: "A mechanism is proposed in which vitamin D inhibits previously initiated melanomas from becoming clinically apparent." Two of the researchers on this study, Frank Garland, PhD and Cedric Garland, PhD, are among the leading researchers on vitamin D (you will sometimes see them referred to as the "Garland brothers" in online articles and blogs).

Melanoma in a Nutshell:

- Only 3 percent of all skin cancers are melanoma.
- Only 20 to 30 percent of melanomas are found in existing moles, while 70 to 80 percent arise on apparently normal skin.
- The risk for developing melanoma for males and females doubles with more than five sunburns.
- An estimated 178,560 cases of melanoma will be diagnosed in the United States in 2018. Of those, 87,290 cases will be in situ (non-invasive) and 91,270 cases will be invasive.
- Invasive melanoma is the fifth most common cancer in men and the sixth most common in women.
- Five-year survival rate is about 99 percent in the United States if detected early. The survival rate falls to 63 percent when the disease reaches the lymph nodes and 20 percent when the disease metastasizes to distant organs.
- Characterized by the uncontrolled growth of pigment-producing tanning cells, melanomas may appear suddenly without warning, but they can also develop from or near a mole (especially moles that have an irregular shape or varying colors).
- Men are almost twice as likely to develop melanoma than women.
- Melanomas most frequently appear on the upper body of men, especially the back or on the lower legs of women, but

can occur anywhere on the body, including areas not exposed to sunlight.

- It is the most common cancer in people twenty-five to twenty-nine years old, especially women, who have had significant sun exposure, including sunburns and sun-bed exposures.
- The overall five-year survival rate for melanoma increased from 49 percent (1950–1954) to 92 percent (1996–2003). *Today the estimated five-year survival rate for African Americans is only 65% versus 91% for light-skinned people.*
- People who have had a basal cell carcinoma are at increased risk of developing melanoma; this is most likely due to sunburns, which are common to both cancers.
- Advanced melanoma can spread to internal organs and bone and may result in death.

More statistics can be found at www.skincancer.org.

Remember: If detected in the early stages, melanoma generally can be treated successfully. Survival rates decline dramatically, however, once the cancer has spread. Currently, the gold standard for determining melanoma risk is thorough clinical evaluation. Anyone at high risk should regularly see a dermatologist for a skin evaluation at least once a year. The following list outlines the major risk factors for melanoma:

Melanoma Risk Factors:

- Family history of melanoma.
- History of severe, blistering sunburns. Light-skin individuals are at highest risk, but those with darker skin can also be affected.
- Five or more sunburns, at any age, double the risk of developing melanoma.

- One or more blistering sunburns in childhood or adolescence doubles the risk of developing melanoma.
- Atypical moles (dysplastic nevi).
- History of using tanning salons.
- Weakened immune system.
- History of a prolonged poor nutrition, devoid of high antioxidant–containing foods, especially vegetables and fruits.
- Previous melanoma.
- Many ordinary moles (more than 50).
- Freckles.
- Socioeconomic status. Melanoma is more prevalent in those who are affluent, possibly because they can afford to vacation or maintain outdoor hobbies such as sailing and skiing. They are also more likely to have access to doctors, including dermatologists and get diagnosed.

Marley's Melanoma: An Example of Skin Cancer in Dark Skin

Though people with darker skin types rarely, if ever, suffer from noticeable sunburns, it does not mean they are immune to melanoma. In fact, because many people believe the myth that their dark skin protects them from the disease, they neither take precautions against it nor do they get a proper diagnosis or treatment for melanoma until it has advanced to the stage where it becomes lethal. Essentially, that is what happened to famed reggae singer Bob Marley, a dark-skinned man from Jamaica who died from malignant melanoma at the age of thirty-six. Initially, Marley's melanoma manifested in his right toe, and it was thought to be caused by a soccer injury. When the sore persisted and would not heal, Marley finally got it checked, only to discover that he had melanoma. It was reported that because of his religious Rastafarian beliefs, he did not have the toe amputated and the melanoma spread to his brain, lungs, and stomach, precipitating his death in 1981. Marley's case is one of the more-famous examples of melanoma occurring in a person of color, but it is not unique. As part of the increased skin cancer rates, which have been rising for the past several decades, researchers are also noting more cases of melanoma in African Americans as well as Hispanics.

Skin Self-Exams and Pre-Cancers: Finding the Warning Signs of Cancer

Now that you know a little about the different forms of skin cancer, you may wonder if you are a candidate for developing it. The good news is that skin cancer is one of the few types of cancer that is visible in its early stages—unlike other forms of cancer that attack internal organs and can grow to a significant size before they are detected. Remember: early detection often equals a high cure rate. In order to take advantage of this characteristic of skin cancer, however, you need to know how to evaluate your body for its warning signs. In this section, you will get basic guidelines to help you recognize the "pre-cancer" condition of actinic keratosis as well as the abnormal-looking moles or suspicious skin areas that could possibly be skin cancer lesions. You'll also find out about the best ways to conduct a skin self-exam.

Moles (or Nevi)

Moles, also known as nevi, are growths on the skin that can be present at birth or grow anytime during life and generally peak in adolescence. Changes in moles during pregnancy are typically normal due to hormonal changes and the skin expansion. However, changes are typically symmetrical, so if there is a question a dermatologist visit is in order. Moles can be flat or raised, are usually round or oval, and are no larger than a pencil eraser. As people age, moles may change in shape and can even disappear. These growths occur when melanocytes (pigment-producing cells) grow in clusters. Colors vary from pink or tan to light beige or brown.

Large moles, including those present at birth, pose the highest risk for malignant changes. Sunburns, particularly those occurring in childhood, are cited as the main cause of moles developing into melanomas. UVB rays have long been singled out as the main risk factor, but more recent studies point to the deep-penetrating UVA rays as also being a causal factor for melanoma. Here is an overview of the two main types of moles that are linked to melanoma:

Dysplastic (Atypical) Nevi: Dysplastic (atypical) nevi are moles with an appearance that differs from common, ordinary moles. These nevi tend to be larger than ordinary moles, with irregular borders and mixed colors. They can be present in large numbers. A dysplastic nevus (which is the term for singular nevi) can give rise to malignant melanoma. Dysplastic nevi are common. A simple dysplastic nevus carries little risk for melanoma and does not identify a person as melanoma prone.

Heredity appears to play a part in the formation of atypical moles, they run in families. Dysplastic nevus-melanoma syndrome refers to the presence of multiple dysplastic nevi and melanoma in two or more first-degree relatives. Patients with this background have a significant increased risk for developing melanoma.

Clark's Nevi: A type of dysplastic nevi, Clark's Nevi, is an atypical mole or moles with features similar to melanoma, including irregular borders, slight variations in color, or asymmetry. Under the microscope, this type of mole has features that are in-between a normal mole and a melanoma. Clark's Nevi is considered pre-cancerous and should be removed.

Skin Self-Examination

Now that you have some idea about what to look for, how are you going to find potential skin cancer sites on your body? One way to discover those problem areas is through a skin self-examination, which is the main tool that can help alert you to potentially troublesome changes in your skin. The most common skin cancers and pre-cancers can be detected on the face and the front of the body. However, the back of the body is difficult to view accurately and small skin cancers or changes in moles will often go unnoticed. I have tried with mirrors to get a better view of moles on my back, and I have concluded that it is nearly impossible. Mainly, it is important to become familiar with your own body and frequently (once a month is advised) inspect your skin. I would also suggest having a friend or family member photograph the back side of your body and include closeups of moles or questionable areas; this history will be helpful to your dermatologist.

Know Your Skin

I examine my face regularly and, at one point, I noticed a tiny white bump under my nose that was not a pimple. I showed it to my dermatologist who did not think it was cancer. He removed it anyway, and it turned out to be a basal cell carcinoma. Finding it so early resulted in two stitches.

The most important criterion in self-diagnosing a potential melanoma is a tool referred to as the "ABCDE rule," which is outlined below. I have seen two examples of what the "E" in this rule stands for from reputable sources, and think they are both relevant, so I include both of them here. The main thing to remember is this: pay special attention to moles, brown spots, birthmarks, rough skin patches, or beauty marks.

Detecting Skin Cancer: The ABCDE Rule:

A = asymmetry: One half of the mole is unlike the other half or the mole is not evenly round.

B = borders or irregular borders: The border is scalloped or poorly defined.

C = colors or irregular colors: The mole or lesion is irregularly colored, ranging from light brown to dark brown, black and sometimes red, blue, or white.

D = diameter: A mole or lesion is suspicious if it is bigger than the size of a pencil eraser.

E = evolving: A mole changes in size, shape, or color.

E = elevation: This is the "height," or elevation, of a mole. Many moles are elevated, but check to see if the elevation is uneven.

The Ugly Duckling Sign: An Early Melanoma Recognition Tool

Another early detection tool can improve early diagnosis, which is critical to the successful treatment of melanoma. This method for detecting skin lesions is based on the concept that certain moles look different compared to surrounding moles; thus, this detection tool is called the "ugly duckling" sign. During examination, both patients and physicians should be looking for lesions that manifest the characteristics described by the ABCDE Rule as well as those that appear to be "ugly ducklings."

Ugly Duckling Examples: To check for "ugly ducklings" note the pattern of moles that you have and see if any do not match the typical pattern. The following guidelines will give you an idea of what to look for:

- Typically, moles have a dominant mole pattern with slight variation in size. The "ugly duckling" may be darker or larger than all other moles.
- There may be two predominant mole patterns, one of larger moles and the other of smaller, darker moles. The "ugly duckling" could be small and lacking pigmentation.
- Moles that feel different from other moles are also suspicious. Most may feel smooth while one "ugly duckling" feels rough, or vice versa.
- An "ugly duckling" may also be an area of skin that feels or looks different, especially if you have noticed changes in a specific area.

Skin Self-Examination Steps

It is a good idea to purchase a magnifying glass to view suspected spots. Circle spots in question and photograph them. Also, photograph moles so you can watch them over time to see if any changes have occurred. Before seeing a dermatologist, you should always do a thorough self-examination. If you have several areas for your dermatologist to check, circle the areas with a washable marker. When my dermatologist examines my skin, he also uses a magnifying glass and takes pictures of questionable areas. Following are some helpful tips for your self-examination:

- Start at the top of the head (scalp) and end with the feet.
- Give special attention to the face, ears, neck, and sun-exposed areas.

- Include the armpits, hands, finger webs, nail beds, and soles of the feet.
- A mirror should be used to examine the back and skin between the buttocks. (This is nearly impossible, so I recommend having someone else look at areas that are hard to view.)
- Note any skin growth that appears pearly, translucent, brown, black, or multicolored. Look also for any scar-like lesions.
- Pay special attention to the borders of moles—irregular borders, variation in color, and any size changes.
- Feel the skin. Rough areas may be actinic keratosis or possible skin cancer.
- Photograph moles for an accurate record of what the moles once looked like. You will need help photographing the back side of your body. This is an excellent way to keep track of any changes, and you can point out areas of concern to your doctor.
- Lesions that itch, change, or bleed, or sores that don't heal, are alarming signals; see your dermatologist.
- Skin cancers of all kinds can also show up as tiny areas at first; they may look like a small new pinkish mole, for instance, or a new indentation that looks like a scar. These skin changes can be serious forms of skin cancer, so pay attention whenever you see a change.

NOTE: some skin cancers and actinic keratosis can appear to come and go; sometimes they will bleed, look like pimples, or itch; and these symptoms may stop and reappear weeks or even months later. Pay careful attention to any skin changes.

Finding a Good Dermatologist

While it is important to regularly examine your skin at home, it is equally important to be examined by a dermatologist. However, a professional examination is not foolproof, which I discovered firsthand. Over the past several years, four dermatologists examined my skin from head to toe, and it surprised me that my experience with each doctor was so different. One doctor in particular offered a very thorough exam, while others seemed to skim over my body. I also discovered that once a diagnosis has been made, the opinions vary from topical treatments to surgery for the same exact lesion.

The lesson I learned is that each of us needs to know the signs of skin cancer and check our own skin. Below are tips for finding and visiting a doctor.

Tips to Finding a Good Doctor: If you are a high-risk candidate, consider having your skin examined by more than one doctor.

- Get a referral from a friend or family member.
- Check websites that specialize in patients who are referring doctors in your area. In the San Francisco Bay area where I live, many of the top doctors are not accepting new patients unless you are a family member, so it can be challenging finding a top doctor.

Preparation for a Doctor's Visit: Before your visit, make sure you go over your own skin. If you suspect any area, point that out to the doctor. If you are suspicious of an area, even if the doctor is not, insist on a biopsy.

- Make notes of any questionable skin areas, as mentioned above.
- Once you are in the office, notice how thorough he/she is examining your skin. Does the doctor use a magnifying glass and a bright light for viewing your skin?

What the Doctor Should Examine: Basically, the doctor should examine your entire body carefully, especially if you are high risk. Make sure the following body areas are included:

- scalp: the doctor should look through your hair
- soles of feet
- fingers and fingernails
- pubic and buttock regions. Some doctors will not examine these areas and instead refer you to your primary care doctor or, for women, your gynecologist.
- face, ears, nose. Make sure to take off your glasses.

While some doctors do not provide a thorough exam, other doctors biopsy too many areas needlessly. When in question, ask for a biopsy. If you have two differing opinions who should you believe? And, for those who have the means a third opinion may be in order.

Eye Cancer and Eye Damage from Sun Exposure

Because your eyes, like your skin, contain melanin-producing cells, it is possible for melanoma to develop in them. Not much evidence exists, however, showing that ultraviolet (UV) radiation from the sun increases the risk of eye melanoma, which is also known as ocular melanoma. While eye melanoma is difficult to detect and may not cause highly noticeable early symptoms, the Mayo Clinic recommends that you check with your doctor if any of these warning signs bothers you:

- a growing dark spot on the iris
- a sensation of flashing lights
- a change in the shape of the pupil (the dark circle) at the center of your eye

- poor or blurry vision in one eye
- loss of vision in the affected eye

In developing a conscious relationship with the sun, however, cancer is not the only concern you should have. Your eyes also need protection to avoid the risk of cataracts. Cataracts develop when the lens of the eye becomes progressively opaque, resulting in blurred vision.

In areas of the world where sun exposure is intense (especially where there is additional sun reflection from sand or water), cataracts are a leading cause of blindness.

Be sure to wear sunglasses in sun-intense situations and brimmed hats to protect your eyes from direct sun exposure. Before full-spectrum sunglasses were invented, sunglasses sometimes caused more eye damage because the pupil of the eye would open and allow UVA rays to penetrate deep into the tissues of the eye. Although there is little proof that sunglasses can prevent eye melanoma, they may reduce the risk of your developing cataracts if the glasses are uniformly dark, block both UVA and UVB rays, and prevent light from the sides from hitting your eyes (as wraparound frames do).

Coping with a Diagnosis of Skin Cancer

Even though skin cancer is highly curable, it can still be frightening to be diagnosed with it—especially melanoma. On top of that, skin cancer is the type of condition that could be the manifestation of behavior you may have engaged in years before the onset of the disease. An avid tanner as a teen might have to deal with skin cancer in middle age (or even younger). But it does little good to regret the things you might have done differently to protect your body from skin cancer. If you or someone in your family does develop skin cancer, it is more productive to take steps to become informed so that you will avail yourself of the best treatment options.

Keep in mind also that there are many proactive steps you can take now to minimize future skin cancers, including sun protection strategies, a heathy lifestyle of good nutrition, and exercise that strengthens the body's response to skin cancer. In the next chapter, you will learn about the various treatment options available for skin cancer.

Key Points from Chapter 9 — When the Sun Is Too Much—Skin Cancer Risks

- Skin cancers are most common on sun exposed areas

- Healthy skin needs to be hydrated

- A diet rich in vegetables and fruit add the needed antioxidants to help protect your skin

- Healthy digestion is important for the skin

- Skin cancer is cured 85 to 99 percent of the time

- Sunburns at any time in life increase the risk of skin cancer

- Having multiple moles and atypical moles increases skin cancer risk

- BCC often referred to as the "friendly cancer" is not so friendly if it develops in sun sensitive areas such as the lips, nose and near the eyes

- Certain medications and herbs can make your skin more sensitive to sun

- Melanoma is curable if caught early and treated early

- Check your skin regularly

Chapter 10

Skin Cancer Treatments, Medical and Alternative

When you or someone close to you is diagnosed with skin cancer, you may have to learn a whole new medical vocabulary. To understand that vocabulary, and to make the best treatment choices, it is important know which type of skin cancer you're dealing with. The following section expands on what we have discussed about the primary categories of skin cancer.

First you will learn about the brief definitions of pre-cancer and the various types of common skin cancers, along with other commonly used medical definitions. The section begins with a refresher on the acronyms used for skin cancer that you will see throughout the rest of this chapter.

AK: actinic keratosis is also referred to as solar keratosis and pre-cancer

BCC: basal cell carcinoma

SCC: squamous cell carcinoma

Melanoma: is not usually abbreviated, but the four sub-types of melanoma each have their own acronyms and are explained below.

Following is an excerpt from skincancer.org: "An actinic keratosis (AK), also known as a solar keratosis, is a crusty, scaly growth caused by damage from exposure to ultraviolet (UV) radiation. You'll often see the plural, *keratoses*, because there is seldom just one. AK is considered a pre-cancer because if left alone, a small percentage of AKs can develop into skin cancer, most commonly, squamous cell carcinoma (SCC)."

Skin Cancer Types and Diagnosis

The National Cancer Institute (NCI) points out the importance of knowing the precise type of cancer with which a patient has been diagnosed because it has a direct impact on medical decisions. According to the NCI, treatment options depend on these four factors:

1. the type of cancer
2. the size and location of the tumor
3. the stage of the cancer (whether it has remained local or has spread deeper into the skin or to other places in the body)
4. the patient's general health

Basal Cell Carcinoma Subtypes and Characteristics

Nodular-ulcerative

This is the most common form of BCC and presents (appears) as a small, pearly dome-shaped papule. Over time the center will indent (ulcerate) and may bleed on and off, and the tumor can grow down to the fat layer of skin where it typically stops and then spreads on top of the fat layer. I had one of these cancers on my arm for years before I realized what it was. When I did recognize it, it was easily excised and required eight stitches. Had it appeared on my face, it would have been much more of a problem and may have required cosmetic surgery, depending on location.

Superficial

This is a fairly common form of BCC, and it is the least aggressive subtype. It tends to remain in the epidermis. Usually it appears as several scaly, dry areas mainly on the trunks, arms, and legs. It will slowly spread if left untreated. Diagnosis can be difficult since superficial BCC also resembles psoriasis, eczema, and actinic keratosis.

Pigmented

This is not a very common form. It is seen more often in people with darker skin color. It looks like the nodular type but will vary in color, due to the melanin, and may be brown, black, or multicolor. Sometimes it can be mistaken for malignant melanoma.

Infiltrative BCC, which also encompasses morpheaform and micronodular BCC, is more difficult to treat with conservative methods, given its tendency to penetrate into deeper layers of the skin. This is not a common form.

Basosquamous

This rare form of skin cancer has characteristics of BCC and SCC and is diagnosed with a biopsy. It can be an aggressive skin cancer that has a higher rate of metastasis.

Squamous Cell Carcinoma

The most common type of SCC is Bowen's disease ("SCC in situ"). Another condition, keratoacanthoma, is sometimes included as a second type of SCC in situ. However, some specialists do not agree that it is a second type but that it is a separate diagnose. That said, both forms are only rarely a threat, but could develop into a more dangerous type if not treated promptly. At times, aggressive SCC can appear like a different form of skin cancer such as BCC. Only a biopsy can help determine the diagnosis.

Bowen's Disease (SCC in situ)

This form of cancer is a very early form of skin cancer that's easily treatable. The main sign is a red, scaly patch on the skin. It may be mistaken for a fungus or a rash. It affects the squamous cells—which are in the outermost layer of skin—and is sometimes referred to as squamous cell carcinoma in situ.

Keratoacanthoma (KA)

This can appear as a cyst or "boil." It manifests as a rapidly forming lump with a central dry, crusty core. It is typically slightly red or a skin color. It is most commonly found on sun-exposed areas, especially the forearms, hands, and face. It is more common in men older than forty-five years of age.

KA may be difficult to distinguish visually from a skin cancer. Under the microscope, it closely resembles SCC. In order to differentiate between the two, almost the entire structure needs to be removed and examined. While some pathologists classify KA as a distinct entity and not a malignancy, about 6 percent of clinical and histological keratoacanthomas do progress to invasive and aggressive squamous cell cancers; some pathologists may label KA as "well-differentiated squamous cell carcinoma, KA variant," and surgery may be recommended.

NOTE: I had one of these develop rapidly on the back of my hand. The first biopsy came back as SCC. My dermatologist had the same biopsy sent to the University of California in San Francisco for a second opinion and it came back keratoacanthoma. Instead of surgery my dermatologist treated it three times with chemo injections. I did not want to risk the 6 percent chance that it would evolve into SCC.

Melanoma Subtypes and Characteristics

Melanoma can be difficult to diagnose. This means that some people who have a melanoma lesion will go undiagnosed, and some people who do not have melanoma will be wrongly diagnosed. Make sure you have up-to-date information regarding diagnosis, typing, staging, and treatment options. Also, it is wise to get a second opinion at a university if possible, for a more precise diagnosis, if you or your doctor have reason to question the results.

NOTE: In 2018 I was diagnosed with a small melanoma on my face. My doctor sent the same biopsy to UCSF and their report was benign.

There are four types of melanoma. Three begin as tumors confined within a site (in situ tumors), usually within the upper portion of the epidermis. If melanoma is caught before metastasis, early-stage prognosis is excellent. Here are more details on each type:

Superficial Spreading Melanoma (SSM): 70 Percent of All Cases

SSM tends to grow slowly, taking up to several years before it is obvious. Its appearance varies from multicolored or dark, raised or flat, with irregular borders and indentations; and it is more frequently found on sun-exposed areas. SSM is the most common subtype of melanoma, accounting for about 70 percent of all cases, particularly between the ages of thirty to fifty. It occurs most frequently on the upper back of men and women as well as the lower extremities of women. It has two stages of development. In the first phase, where it can stay for months to years, prognosis is excellent. If it grows to a phase two, it can turn into a dangerous malignancy.

Nodular Melanoma (NM): 10 to 15 Percent

Rapid growth is the hallmark of NM, which typically is aggressive. It tends to appear in normal skin rather than moles or lesions or a pre-existing lesion. By the time it is discovered, it is often fairly advanced. The average age of onset is fifty-three years. It appears most commonly on light-skinned people on areas that have frequently been exposed to the sun, including the trunk, arms, legs, head, and neck (especially the scalp in men). The nodule may be black, brown, blue, gray, tan, or even red. It tends to be round, with smooth and irregular borders. About 5 percent lack pigment (amelanotic melanoma). Despite its aggressive nature, if caught early prognosis is good.

Acral Lentiginous Melanoma (ALM): Approximately 2 to 3 Percent

ALM is the most common melanoma in Asians and people with dark skin. It is referred to as the "hidden melanoma" because it appears on areas of the body that are not easily examined or noticed. It can appear in nail beds, palms, soles of the feet, and mucous membranes. On average, it is primarily seen on people older than sixty-five years of age, but it has equal gender distribution. It may be multicolored, but more frequently it is brown or black, with irregular borders, and flat or nodular. This type of melanoma is aggressive and usually advanced at diagnosis. It may appear as a blood blister or bruise and could possibly have a streaked appearance. ALM does not seem to be related to sun exposure.

Lentigo Maligna and Lentigo Maligna Melanoma (LMM): Approximately 5 Percent

This type of *in situ* melanoma is found most often in the elderly, arising on chronically sun-exposed, damaged skin on the face, ears, arms, and upper trunk. Lentigo maligna is the most common form of melanoma in Hawaii. When this cancer becomes invasive, it is referred to as lentigo maligna melanoma.

The lesion is flat and varies in color: tan, brown, black, or other colors. The borders can be scalloped and convoluted on the surface skin layer. LMM can grow fairly large—3 centimeters and more. It does not tend to metastasize as some other melanomas do and, therefore, with removal there is an excellent prognosis.

Stages of Melanoma

Melanoma is also categorized into stages. One system that is used for melanoma staging is the tumor, node, metastasis (TNM) system. The early stages of melanoma, stages 0 to 2, do not involve lymph nodes or metastasis. Eighty-five percent of melanoma cases are diagnosed in the early stages. These early stages are local (more superficial) lesions that have not metastasized and are typically treated with surgery. The cure rate is very high, 95 to 99 percent. This underscores the importance of early detection and treatment.

Melanoma stages are assigned based on the size or thickness of the tumor, whether or not it has spread to the lymph nodes or other organs, and certain other characteristics, such as growth rate.

TNM Staging

The American Joint Commission on Cancer has developed a uniform staging system that allows doctors to determine how advanced a melanoma is, and to share that information with each other in a meaningful way. This melanoma staging system, known as TNM staging, is composed of three key pieces of information:

- **Tumor (T)** describes the tumor's thickness, or how deep it has grown into the skin. The thickness of the melanoma, also known as the Breslow measurement, is an important factor in predicting whether or not a tumor has spread. The thicker the melanoma, the greater the chance of it spreading. The rate at which the tumor cells are dividing (also known as the mitotic rate), and the presence or absence of ulceration (an open, bleeding sore), are also considered in determining the T category.

- **Nodes (N)** indicates whether or not the melanoma cancer has spread to nearby lymph nodes, or the channels connecting the lymph nodes.
- **Metastasis (M)** refers to whether the melanoma has spread to distant organs, as well as on levels of lactate dehydrogenase (LDH), a substance in the blood.

Melanoma may be staged before surgery (clinical staging), based on physical exam and imaging results. It will also be staged after surgery (pathologic staging), in which the clinical information will be combined with information gained from biopsies. Because it uses more information, pathologic cancer staging is the most accurate.

If you have been diagnosed with melanoma, several excellent websites can help you understand the proper diagnosis and make sure your lesion has been properly staged. For up-to-date staging information check the Melanoma Foundation website at aimat-melanoma.org. The Cancer Treatments of America website, www.cancercenter.com/melanoma/stages offers a staging tool that will guide you through questions to help you identify the correct stage of melanoma. Two other helpful websites are WebMD (webmd.com /melanoma-skin-cancer) and http://melanomainternational.org.

Stage 0 melanoma involves the epidermis (outer skin layer), but the lesion has not reached the underlying dermis. This stage is also called melanoma in situ.

Stage I melanoma is characterized by tumor thickness and may or may not have ulceration. There is no evidence of regional lymph node or distant metastasis (spreading).

Stage II melanoma is also characterized by tumor thickness and ulceration status. There is no evidence of regional lymph node or distant metastasis.

Stage III melanoma is characterized by the level of regional lymph node involvement. There is no evidence of distant metastasis.

Stage IV melanoma has traveled beyond the regional lymph nodes to more distant areas of the body. The most common sites of metastasis are vital organs and soft tissue.

Trudy's Story: This story was sent to me by a friend and colleague, Trudy Mestermacher, PhD. It illustrates just how virulent a simple change on the lips can be.

Being a holistic doctor, I have had a mind-set of preventative, natural ways of living my life. Though I also have had to deal with an elderly father who has had many skin cancers that had to be removed and which he most likely got from being a contractor in the 1950s through the 1960s, I never expected that I would get skin cancer—and a serious form of cancer in a highly vulnerable location!

In early April 2018, however, I noticed a small white flat pimple located on my right lower lip. I saw my dermatologist in early May and after she took a measurement, she said, "Let's see if it is larger in three weeks." For a few days, I thought it was just a normal white pimple, and I was going to wait until my dermatologist saw me again. When I noticed, however, how this white spot was starting to get to the lip line, I decided to get a second dermatologist's opinion on May 11. A biopsy was taken that same day. One week later, it came back squamous cell carcinoma. On May 18, I had the stitches from the biopsy removed. On May 23, I underwent an eight-hour surgery with another doctor to remove a 2.5-centimeter skin cancer.

It took four separate cuttings of the doctor coming back to get more tissue from my lip before the surgeon said he finally had removed all the cancer cells from the lip. For each separate cutting in the Mohs surgery, the surgeon cut out additional tissue and then examined that tissue to see if all the margins were clear of cancer cells. When my surgeon was finished, one third of my lower lip and an area of tissue the size of a half dollar was gone.

To close the huge hole in my lip, he brought in another surgeon, so they could discuss which would be the best option. They both agreed a "wedge" cut into my chin down to my jaw line and also a "wedge cut" on the inside of my lip down into my gums would be the best way to cosmetically close up the area. This would require about forty to fifty more injections of anesthetic into my chin after the thirty to forty injections I had already received for the cancer and tissue removal.

At 4:30, I left the building with an appointment to see an oncologist. The surgeon's report said he had removed all of the cancer and cleared the margins, but he had to take enough tissue to remove some cancer cells that had intruded into some nerves—and this fact might require further treatment. The oncologist recommended radiation to try to prevent the possibility that the cancer would return. Since lip skin is not like regular skin cancer in that it can more readily return to the lip, or mouth, or jaw area, and since there had been some nerve intrusion, radiation was the best way to destroy any rogue cells that might be in the area. I was therefore referred to a radiologist.

After six weeks of healing from five layers of stitches in my jaw, gums, and lip, I started six weeks of radiation. My radiologist had previous experience treating other lip cancer patients. He made a plastic mold to go around a lead shield that would be placed in front of my teeth and behind my lip to protect my jaw bone and teeth.

After five weeks of treatment, I was experiencing such phenomenal pain and swelling of my lip and chin from the radiation, that radiation was stopped for a few days. I then finished that sixth week with an increased dose of radiation and a reduced radiation field, which focused radiation on the scar area of my chin. I completed my radiation on August 24 and have watched the redness, pain, and swelling subside.

All my doctors said that my lip skin cancer most likely resulted from sun exposure. Not being one who spent time trying to get a suntan, I just couldn't see how I ended up with skin cancer—especially on the lower lip.

What have I realized as a result of all this? Even though you may have increased or even high vitamin D3 levels and you may not be a "sun worshiper," skin cancer can develop in unexpected places. Therefore, you must not only constantly guard against unnecessary exposure to the sun, but also have suspicious spots on your skin checked early! Our immune system ages along with us and cannot destroy cancer cells as readily as when we are younger.

Treating the Whole Patient

Understanding skin cancer types and treatment options is necessary when you're dealing with a cancer diagnosis. But during that process, it can be easy to get caught up in searching for the one single treatment that will cure the problem or make it all go away. In that single-minded focus, however, we often lose sight of the bigger picture. Cancer, in particular, demands that we take care of our bodies in a holistic way—getting proper rest, eating a healthy diet, and gathering emotional support. And though the vast majority of skin cancers are not life threatening, they can give us a wake-up call to take better care of ourselves and make a commitment to staying healthy.

Among the various types of cancer that can arise in the body, skin cancers have one of the highest survival rates of all cancers. Even melanoma, the most serious form of skin cancer, has a five-year survival rate of 95 to 99 percent when it is treated in the earliest stages. However, the survival rate falls to 63 percent when it reaches the lymph nodes and 20 percent when it metastasizes to distant organs.

Keep in mind that skin cancer accounts for only one percent of all cancer deaths. Understanding the diagnosis and knowing your options can help reduce the fear and worry that may come up if you or a loved one is diagnosed with skin cancer.

Medical treatment options for skin cancer range from superficial surgeries and topical creams, to the less commonly used radiation and chemotherapy for the more serious forms. These therapies may be combined, and each approach has its advantages and disadvantages.

Meanwhile, alternative health-care providers may advise you to fight skin cancer by using specially formulated salves or herbs, which may, in some cases, seem to be successful. Although I am a supporter, proponent, and practitioner of alternative medicine, I also recognize that, unfortunately, unconventional treatments often do not have rigorous studies to back up their claims, and they also can have side effects and contraindications, just as standard medical treatments do. In addition, skin cancer (as you learned in the last chapter) can present with varying degrees of severity—from superficial non-malignant basal cell carcinoma to life-threatening melanoma.

Medical options depend on the specifics of the diagnosis and the type of skin cancer being treated. To help you determine the best options (for yourself or someone else) following is an overview of different skin cancer treatments and medications available today. In addition, I'll share some of my own personal experiences with conventional as well as alternative treatments. In general, standard skin cancer treatments are performed on an outpatient basis, often in a dermatologist's office or clinic. Below you will find many treatment options for skin cancer and pre-cancerous skin lesions. There is a section specifically on pre-cancer following all the treatment options for skin cancer. Since surgery is one of the predominant forms of conventional treatment for certain skin cancers, we'll examine this option first.

Medical Treatment Options for Skin Cancers

Cauterization or diathermy (Curettage and cautery)

Curettage (scraping) and cautery (heat) is used to treat some BCCs and SCC in situ. Also, used to treat Bowen's Disease.

1. Surgical Removal

When doctors surgically excise—that is, cut out—tumor growths from the skin, they may use scalpels, laser beams, or electrosurgery, among other tools and techniques. Once removed, the suspected cancer specimen is sent to a lab (or possibly examined on the spot) to verify that malignant cells have been completely removed. Usually, a border of healthy skin around the tumor growth that will be removed to improve the odds of eliminating all of the cancer cells. Dermatologists, surgeons, or possibly radiation oncologists may perform the following types of surgery in treating skin cancer:

Mohs Surgery: This procedure is the most accurate for treating and removing BCC and SCC. This micrographic surgery is named after its originator, Dr. Frederick Moh. In preparation for it, the surgery is carefully mapped so that only the tumor area is removed. Once under way, the doctor cuts away the skin growth layer by layer and then immediately views the tissue under a microscope to make sure the margins are clear of any residual cancer. This procedure allows the doctor to remove the smallest amount of healthy tissue, and it ultimately leaves a smaller scar (which can be an important consideration when a skin cancer site is located on the face). Mohs is used by some surgeons for certain melanomas, but the technique is not accepted by all physicians.

Although Mohs can be performed on an outpatient basis, patients may need to be in the doctor's office for four to eight hours while a pathology report is prepared. Further, because of the skill level required, it is best to seek a practitioner who is specially trained in this procedure. While there are many Moh's surgeons in my area my dermatologist only recommends two, since these doctors have years of experience and the best outcomes, including cosmetic appearance.

Melanoma always requires surgery. Surgery typically involves the removal of more healthy tissue as a precaution. How much healthy tissue is removed will depend on the stage of melanoma. For more advanced cases of melanoma, surgery to remove the skin lesion and medications including chemotherapy may be recommended to stop the spread of the disease.

In recent years, Mohs micrographic surgery, which many physicians consider the most effective technique for removing BCC and SCC, has been increasingly used as an alternative to standard excision for certain melanomas. Keep in mind that doctors must specialize in Mohs and if they do not, this option may not be offered to you.

Excisional Surgery: This basic form of surgery is different from Mohs surgery for skin cancer. Instead of removing layers of the lesion, the surgeon will cut out the entire skin growth and its surrounding border of normal tissue. The tissue then goes to a laboratory, so it can be checked to see if any cancer cells remain. This form of surgery usually takes with it more healthy tissue to ensure complete removal. I had this one done on one BCC where I did not care about a scar, and I was left with eight stitches and a scar that is barely visible.

Electrodesiccation and Curettage: In this procedure, which is most often used for small or thin basal cell carcinomas, the doctor will first numb the area to be treated and remove most of the cancer growth. Then the doctor will scrape away layers of cancer cells with a sharp, spoon-shaped tool called a curette. To control bleeding and remove any remaining cancer cells, an electric current is sent through the treated area. A small, flat, white or light-colored scar may remain after this procedure.

Cryotherapy/Liquid Nitrogen Treatment ("Freezing"): Cryotherapy is the use of liquid nitrogen to destroy a lesion.

Cryotherapy may be a good option for benign lesions, such as actinic keratosis. It is sometimes used treat thin, superficial BCC. Cryotherapy should be when there are only a few lesions to treat, and the lesions have clear borders.

Laser Surgery: Instead of using a traditional scalpel, doctors may employ a precise, intense beam of light to destroy cancer cells. Most commonly, this form of surgery is used for growths on the outermost layer of skin.

> The thought of having your nose, eyelid, or lips diagnosed with skin cancer should be a serious incentive to vigilantly protect these areas.

NOTE: One of the disadvantages of laser surgery, cryosurgery, or electrodesiccation and curettage is that the margins around the skin growth are not available for examination. This means it is difficult to determine if all of the cancerous cells have been removed.

Now that we have learned about the available surgical treatments for skin cancer we will now learn about additional treatment options.

2. Immunotherapy

Immunotherapy is also called biologic therapy because, essentially, it taps into the biological processes of the body to ward off disease. This approach stimulates the body's natural immune system to fight cancer and, in some cases, to lessen the side effects of certain treatments. While chemotherapy works to poison cancer cells or stop those cells from dividing and growing, immunotherapy marshals the body's own ability to eliminate or "reject" cells that pose a danger to the body. In the case of skin cancer, immunotherapy simulates the body to target and kill cancer cells.

In medical circles, it is one of the most exciting forms of treatment on the horizon, as new protocols are being tested in clinical trials, and some immunotherapy drugs are already being used against skin cancer and other forms of cancer. For instance, interferon alfa-2b is currently in use against melanoma that has spread to the lymph nodes, while interleukin-2 is being tested for melanoma treatment. The *New England Journal of Medicine* reported that the drug ipilimumab improved the survival rate of patients who had advanced melanoma.

Aldara and generic Zyclara cream is an FDA-approved topical medication used to treat actinic keratosis and *superficial* basal cell carcinoma. Both medications contain the active ingredient imiquimod. Although it is sometimes listed along with other topical chemotherapy treatments, it is not a chemotherapeutic agent. Common side effects are redness, peeling of the skin, itching, flaking, and possible blistering. Aldara stimulates local production of interferon and cytokines and treats the lesion from the inside out. Some patients report uncomfortable oozing sores. If you experience a severe reaction, call your doctor. Patients must be informed about how to use this cream correctly, including when to remove it, since the surrounding healthy skin can be irritated. If applied correctly that reaction should not be a problem for most people. Aldara is used two to five times per week for six to sixteen weeks. The exact amount of time will depend on the condition you are treating. Personally, I would not treat a superficial BCC on my face with Aldara because superficial BCC can look very much like other BCC, such as infiltrative.

TIP:

Make sure you understand the extent of the normal skin reaction to anticipate. If you experience more than that, consult with your doctor.

NOTE: I used Aldara on a superficial basal cell carcinoma on my shoulder. It worked beautifully with only minimal redness and soreness. After six weeks, the BCC was gone. I had no scarring, leaving the treated area looking perfectly normal. However, I have also known people who experienced extreme reactions to Aldara.

3. Chemotherapy—Topical

Chemotherapy is often thought of as a cancer treatment that comes in the form of pills or injections. The rationale for chemotherapy is that it delivers anticancer drugs to the body in order to destroy cancer cells, and people are generally aware that it can cause significant (horrible for some) side effects such as nausea, impaired brain function, and weight loss. For some skin cancers that have not metastasized, the fundamental approach for chemotherapy is the same as for other cancers—but instead of being taken internally (as with "systemic chemotherapy"), the drugs are applied to the surface of the skin, or topically, thus the term, *topical chemotherapy*. It is prescribed to patients as a cream or lotion, which is applied to the skin a couple of times a day for a period of weeks. The symptoms are usually only discomfort at the site where the cream is administered.

Fluorouracil (Efudex, Carac 5-FU) is a chemotherapy cream that can be used to treat actinic keratosis as well as very small SSC or BCCs. 5-FU cream is applied regularly for two to three weeks, and it can cause significant redness (inflammation), itching, and erosion of the skin. (These conditions usually resolve two or more weeks after the completion of treatment.) The skin often appears normal after treatment, with little or no scarring.

4. Photodynamic Therapy

This treatment destroys skin cancer cells by subjecting them to drugs that increase their sensitivity to light. Once the photosensitizing

drug is selectively absorbed by the tumor (and after an "incuba-
tion" period that can last several minutes or days), the tumor area is
exposed to a strong light, which kills the cancerous cells.

When used to treat cancer growths near the skin's surface, this
treatment may leave less scarring than surgical techniques. It may,
however, also be less effective than surgery in preventing recur-
rences of skin cancer.

Porfimer sodium has been approved for the treatment of some
skin cancers such as basal cell carcinoma and squamous cell carcinoma. Photodynamic therapy (PDT) is an emerging treatment for
skin cancer and has many benefits with few downsides. For up-to-
date information visit www.skincancer.org.

5. Electrochemotherapy (ETC) Gene Therapy

Experimental procedures with gene therapy may also offer some
promise for melanoma patients. One technique, electroporation,
uses electrical current to "shock" a tumor, causing pores to form
within it. Those pores make the tumor more receptive to injections of an immune-boosting gene. This is another exciting and
quickly evolving treatment option. Patients treated with ECT for
some types of melanoma showed that their tumors did not reoccur.
Some research is supporting the use of ETC for melanoma, though
more research is needed.

6. Radiation

Radiation therapy, which can often be effectively employed
against tumors in the brain or lungs, is not commonly used to treat
skin cancer. It may, however, be offered as an option for treating
very large or inoperable skin cancer growths, as well as those that
have spread to the lymph nodes, or for small tumors located on
the eyelid, ears, or nose. This form of therapy may be used to treat

the rare instances of significant basal or squamous cell carcinomas, lesions, and rarely, melanoma.

Treatment Options for Pre-cancers or Actinic Keratosis (AK)

There are several treatment options for AK. Treatment options will depend on where it is located and how significant the lesions appear. Following is a list of treatment options from the website skincancer.org.

- Cryosurgery: (freezing with liquid nitrogen): this is one of the best treatments for simple types of AK. Some doctors use a spray can of liquid nitrogen and spray the area. Some doctors prefer using a Q-tip to be more precise. After a few days, a scab will form and drop off. This treatment can leave white spots.

- Curettage and desiccation: the physician scrapes or shaves off part or all of the lesion, then applies heat or a chemical agent to stop the bleeding and potentially kill any remaining AK cells.

- Dermabrasion: a skin-resurfacing procedure that uses a rotating device to sand the outer layers of skin. After the procedure, the skin that grows back is usually smoother and younger looking.

- Topical Medications: topical fluorouracil (FU), imiquimod, ingenol mebutate, diclofenac, and chemical peels (trichloro-acetic acid).

- Laser Surgery: the physician uses intense light to vaporize AK tissue.

- Photodynamic Therapy (PDT): especially useful for wide-spread lesions on the face and scalp. The physician applies a light-sensitizing topical agent to the lesions, then uses a strong light to activate the topical agent, destroying the AKs while sparing healthy tissue.

Field Therapy

If you have numerous or widespread actinic keratoses, your doctor may prescribe a topical cream, gel, or solution. These can treat visible and invisible lesions with a minimal risk of scarring. Doctors sometimes refer to this type of therapy as "field therapy," since the topical treatments can cover a wide field of skin as opposed to targeting isolated lesions. I have discussed this approach with dermatologists. Some doctors do not recommend it.

Now that we have covered the medical options for treating pre-cancers and skin cancers let's look at the alternative treatment options to treat these lesions, as well as what you can do to prevent future lesions.

Alternative Skin Cancer Treatments and Skin Care

The field of cancer treatments has long been filled with stories of miracle cures and anecdotal evidence about the success of unconventional treatments. In regard to skin cancer, specifically, you can find any number of websites with testimonials promoting the effectiveness of various salves and creams. Ideally, clinical studies of alternative treatments for skin cancer would help us determine whether or not the recommended product or substance has merit.

People also have home remedies that they have used on their animals and themselves. However, are these older, traditional treatments as good or better than what modern medicine offers? Cancer is a dangerous area to try something that does not have significant studies authenticating its successful use. Add to this that some treatments may remove part of the cancer but leave the remaining cancer growing beneath the surface.

I am personally interested in home remedies; I would like to find something effective that I can use at home, which might save me from medical treatments, including surgery. So, I wish I could enthusiastically recommend alternative treatments for skin cancer. But in my research for this book, and from personal experience with a home treatment, I have decided that when it comes to skin cancer removal, I will head to a good dermatologist. Skin cancer is serious business, so, if you have been diagnosed, investigate reliable sources regarding your options before deciding on treatment. And if nothing else, remember this: have suspicious areas biopsied first—before committing to a treatment plan.

During the course of writing this book, I interviewed many people who eagerly told me that they cured their skin cancer with a home remedy. One even said that she had had melanoma. However, none of them had a biopsy to prove that it was skin cancer to begin with. Do not trust personal testimonials regarding skin cancer treatments.

In the following sections, you will learn about alternative and home treatments for skin cancer.

1. Cancer Salves

The most common and popular online treatment for skin cancer is cancer salve, which has gained popularity with Internet testimonials. It may be called any of these common names: black salve, escharotics, escharotic therapy, botanical salve, Curaderm, and Cansema. These salves may also be known as "escharotics" because they form a scab called an "eschar" on the skin. They contain a variety of herbs added to a base of oils, beeswax, and other ingredients. The active ingredients are usually bloodroot, zinc chloride, or both, while some salves may contain chemicals—all of which can cause a corrosive action. Proponents state that the salve will act only on cancer cells while leaving healthy cells unscathed.

Cancer salves are applied to the skin cancer for a period of weeks. Over time, the salve "eats away" at the cancer, eventually resulting in the eschar (or scab) dropping off of the body. Depending on the appearance of the tissue underneath the wound (after the eschar comes off), another round of salve application may or may not be necessary.

Following is an excerpt from Memorial Sloan Kettering Cancer Center: "Bloodroot is a perennial flowering plant native to eastern North America. It is thought to have antiseptic, cathartic, diuretic, emetic, and escharotic (scab-forming) properties and has been used for inflammation, cough, infections, as an antiplaque agent, and for cancer treatment. The major constituent of bloodroot is sanguinarine, an alkaloid that exhibits antimicrobial, tumoricidal, anticancer, antiangiogenic, and antimicrotubule properties. However, its efficacy has not been tested in humans.

Topical use of bloodroot for skin cancer can lead to severe adverse effects, including disfigurement. The use of sanguinarine as an oral antiplaque agent has been linked to leukoplakia. Bloodroot is an ingredient in black salve, which is promoted as an alternative cancer treatment."

In one of the few research reports on this type of treatment, the *Archives of Dermatological Research* published a study (December 2002) on a handful of patients who decided to self-treat with cancer salves. At least one of the patients was scarred severely after using a bloodroot paste. And, although a couple of these patients seemed to have gotten rid of their tumors or growths, their skin cancers recurred, and they eventually had to undergo extensive surgery.

The American Cancer Society warns people against this form of treatment and offers these cautionary statements on its website:

"All claims that cancer salves cure cancer are based on anecdotal reports and testimonials. There is no scientific evidence that cancer salves cure cancer or any other disease."

"There have been numerous reports of severe scarring and burns associated with the use of cancer salves, and the FDA does not regulate them. The contents of different cancer salves vary and can contain potentially dangerous substances. Women who are pregnant or breast-feeding should NEVER use cancer salves."

One 2017 study, reviewing an ingredient from black salve (sanguinarine) treatments, puts it this way, "However, in vitro studies of sanguinarine suggest it causes indiscriminate destruction of healthy and cancerous tissue . . . It is vital that members of the public are aware of the potential effects and toxicity of commercial salve products."

Bottom line: I do not recommend cancer salves for the treatment of skin cancer.

Cancer Salves: My Story

Many websites are devoted to miraculous stories regarding cancer salves and their ability to cure skin cancer, with dramatic "before" and "after" photos of cancer treatments and personal testimonials attesting to the curative nature of salves. After reading a significant number of testimonials, I was curious enough to investigate these claims. In the late 1990s, I read a book by Ingrid Naiman, entitled *Cancer Salves*. It promoted the idea of cancer salves as an alternative treatment option for skin cancers and, apparently, any cancer. I read the book and also talked directly with Ingrid regarding the use of cancer salves. In reading the book, it was easy to imagine that something topical could treat skin cancer, but its claims about using salves to treat brain cancer was a huge conceptual stretch. According to the book, salves can be applied to the skin over a tumor that is deep in the body and it will pull or "draw out" the cancer from the body.

Prior to my conversation with Ingrid, I had tried a salve from a company other than hers, as an experiment. Their website was laden with testimonials regarding this product, and I spoke with the owner by phone. After using their product for one week, however, literally nothing happened to my skin, fortunately. I shared this information with Ingrid, who said she was not surprised and felt that I would likely have more luck with her product. Perhaps I just got tired of it all, but rather than trying another salve, I decided to have the cancer surgically removed, which was quick and easy in my case.

Since I had only my own experience with cancer salves and no other research to go on at that time, I decided to call herbalist Karyn Sanders, who at the time was the host of *The Herbal Highway*, a weekly show on radio station KPFA in Berkeley, California. Her opinion was not favorable regarding the use of cancer salves; she reported that she had seen several people with gaping wounds who were looking for additional remedies to heal the area treated by the salves. Her main concern regarding salves is that there is no way of knowing if the treated cancers have been fully removed. Also, cancers can tend to grow in areas of irritation, and the salves themselves cause major irritation. Herbs can certainly help the body fight cancer, but Sanders prefers to work in conjunction with medical doctors she trusts. I agreed with her then, and I still agree today. Working with a reputable and competent dermatologist to remove skin cancer growths is the best approach because it is effective and does not involve the risk of leaving cancerous cells or severe deformities that can result from the use of cancer salves.

NOTE: There is one other part to this story you should know about. When I read Ingrid Naiman's book on cancer salves in the 1990s, it featured a cover endorsement by Dr. Andrew Weil (the well-known author of books on integrative medicine), who at one point reported using bloodroot paste on his dog. In 2006, however, when he answered a question on his website regarding the use of bloodroot to treat skin cancer, he advised against it with this statement: "I do not recommend using bloodroot paste, or anything else for that matter, for the self-treatment of skin cancers. It might not get all malignant tissue. Only examination by biopsy can confirm a diagnosis or a cure."

2. Glycoalkaloids

Glycoalkaloids exfoliate the skin. There are alternative doctors supporting this substance as a safe way to remove some skin cancers. The well-known health products promoter Dr. Joseph Mercola ran an article in 2011 titled, "Stunning New Way to Flush Away Skin Cancer." In this article, he promoted the use of topical glycoalkaloid creams to treat skin cancer. There are some studies that show that glycoalkaloids may treat some skin cancers. How exactly does your alternative doctor know how to diagnose skin cancers properly? Some products may treat the surface area of a skin cancer, while leaving the deeper lesion to continue to grow and spread. I do not recommend self-treatment of skin cancer with products that you can buy online. It is impossible to know exactly what is in these products and exactly what they will do.

Apple cider vinegar

I have read about many well-meaning parents treating their children's skin ailments with apple cider vinegar, including potential cancers. In a 2015 paper, dermatologists treated a 14-year-old girl who had applied several drops of vinegar to a mole over the course of three days. Although her mole did peel off, she was also left with skin damage, which could lead to scarring. Perhaps more importantly, she had now made it nearly impossible for the doctors to tell if the mole was cancerous or precancerous.

Besides the home treatments already mentioned, there are other home treatments you will read about on the Internet, including baking soda and coconut oil paste, oils from raspberry seed, frankincense and myrrh, iodine, and vitamin C.

I strongly recommend seeing a dermatologist regarding any suspicious moles or skin changes rather than relying on a testimonial from the Internet.

Feed Your Skin Through Nutrition and Exercise

Good nutrition and safe sun practices are our best weapons against developing future skin cancers. The most important at-home treatment we can do for our skin is to make sure it is getting the nutrients that it needs. The foods that we consume strengthen or weaken our skin. Exercise is also critical for skin health as it improves circulation to and from the skin. When we improve circulation, we bring much-needed nutrients to the skin while removing toxins at the same time.

It is difficult to prove that a given diet or nutrient will slow the growth of an existing cancer. What is known is that certain nutrients support skin health and may prevent certain forms of skin cancer. Fruits and especially vegetables are high in cancer-fighting antioxidants. A healthy, well-balanced diet will boost the body's immune system and give it what it needs to mount a fight against an existing cancer, as well. And, certain lifestyle issues are harmful to the skin, such as smoking and drinking too much alcohol.

Recent research has demonstrated that some antioxidants do indeed promote healthy skin. More dermatologists than ever now advise patients to feast on foods high in these nutrients. Many also suggest applying topical products containing them. The evidence that these compounds prevent skin cancers is stronger for some than others. Following is a list of antioxidants and what foods contain them.

Beta Carotene: Orange-colored vegetables and fruits, including carrots, squash, sweet potatoes, cantaloupe, apricots and mangoes

Lycopene: Tomatoes, watermelon, guava, papaya, apricots, pink grapefruit, blood oranges and other foods

Vitamin C: Oranges, lemons, limes, strawberries, raspberries and certain vegetables, including leafy greens, broccoli and bell peppers

Omega-3 Fatty Acids: Fatty fish such as salmon, sardines, mackerel, herring and albacore tuna, walnuts, flaxseed, chia and hemp seeds

Polyphenols in Tea: Black or green tea has long been regarded as an aid to good health, and many believe it can help reduce the risk of cancer. Most studies of tea and cancer prevention have focused on green tea. The tea polyphenols have been found in animal studies to inhibit tumorigenesis at different organ sites, including the skin, and other organs such as the lung, stomach, and colon. Polyphenols are natural, organic chemicals that are abundant in plant products.

Vitamin D: Sensible sun-exposure, fatty fish such as salmon, mackerel and tuna are excellent sources as well, and you can get small amounts in egg yolks, beef liver and cheese. Cod-liver oil is not recommended as mentioned in Chapter 8. As you have learned it is most important to make sure your vitamin D level is above 40 ng/mL.

Zinc: Oysters, beef, chicken leg, lean pork chops, firm tofu, natto, tempeh, squash and pumpkin seeds, pine nuts and cashews, lentils, beans, yogurt and gouda cheese, oats, shiitake mushrooms, green beans and spinach

Selenium: Brazil nuts and meats such as chicken and grass-fed beef

Vitamin E: Almonds and other nuts, sunflower and other seeds, spinach, soybeans and wheat germ

Tomatoes and Skin Cancer

Many studies have reported that the carotenoids in tomatoes appear to reduce sunburn and may prevent some skin cancers. An Ohio State University study in 2017 reported the following, which is quoted below:

A diet rich in tomatoes cuts skin cancer in half in mice.

Daily tomato consumption appeared to cut the development of skin cancer tumors by half in a mouse study at The Ohio State University. The new study of how nutritional interventions can alter the risk for skin cancers appeared online in the journal *Scientific Reports.*

It found that male mice fed a diet of 10 percent tomato powder daily for 35 weeks, then exposed to ultraviolet light, experienced, on average, a 50 percent decrease in skin cancer tumors compared to mice that ate no dehydrated tomato.

The theory behind the relationship between tomatoes and cancer is that dietary carotenoids, the pigmenting compounds that give tomatoes their color, may protect skin against UV light damage, said Jessica Cooperstone, co-author of the study and a research scientist.

Previous human clinical trials suggest that eating tomato paste over time can dampen sunburns, perhaps thanks to carotenoids from the plants that are deposited in the skin of humans after eating and may be able to protect against UV light damage.

"Lycopene, the primary carotenoid in tomatoes, has been shown to be the most effective antioxidant of these pigments," Cooperstone said.

"However, when comparing lycopene administered from a whole food (tomato) or a synthesized supplement, tomatoes appear more effective in preventing redness after UV exposure, suggesting other compounds in tomatoes may also be at play."

Skin Hydration

Our bodies are about 50 to 65 percent liquid. Water is essential for the health of our skin and for the health of the entire body. Well-hydrated skin looks and feels healthy. As we age, our skin loses the ability to retain moisture. We can slow that process through proper nutrition and skin care. Hydrating the body throughout the day will maximize the moisture in your skin. By now you know that the most popular soda drinks are unhealthy and should be eliminated from your home and are not a good source of liquid.

We do get some liquid from the foods we eat. During the day we need to drink water or herbal teas for the most benefit. We will retain some water from caffeinated drinks; however, caffeine dehydrates the body as does alcohol. How much you need depends on many environmental factors and your personal health. Basically, most people need between six to eight cups of water daily. Some people need more, especially larger people or if you sweat a lot for any reason. Just make sure you drink plenty throughout the day.

Bottomline for healthy Skin

- Hydration: Healthy skin needs to be hydrated. Make sure you are consuming enough water each day.

- Whole foods diet: Minimize or eliminate processed carbohydrates and sugar.

- A diet rich in vegetables and fruit will add the needed antioxidants to help protect your skin.

- Healthy digestion is important for the skin; in fact, when people have a skin condition such as eczema, rosacea, or other skin conditions, quite often there is a digestive problem that may be impacting the condition. Digestive problems, poor food choices, or food sensitivities can exacerbate or cause just about any skin condition.

Now that we can appreciate the benefits of nutrition and exercise to promote healthy skin, we will learn about topical sunscreen protection and sun protection strategies.

Key Points from Chapter 10— Skin Cancer Treatments

- Mohs Surgery is the most accurate for treating and removing BCC and SCC

- Melanoma always requires surgery.

- Cryotherapy or freezing is approved by the FDA for BCC, however the success rate is not as good as Moh's—a consideration when BCC is on the face

- Buying products online to treat skin cancer is not recommended

■ Alternative treatments for skin cancer may only treat the surface of the skin cancer and months later a larger lesion can emerge

■ Feed your skin with a healthy lifestyle

■ A diet high in antioxidants has been shown to reduce sunburns

Chapter 11

Sensible Sun Exposure and Sun Protection

If you were to follow some of the more alarmist advice about sun exposure, you might believe you should never, ever let a single ray of sunshine touch your body. Appreciation for the sun, which was once an object of worship, has sunk to the level of being labeled a "carcinogen."

Yet, as you have been learning in this book, the sun can also provide you with one of the most important nutrients your body needs: vitamin D. Ironically, the same people who advocate avoiding the sun because it could produce skin cancer will also advise to load up on sunscreen—without addressing the carcinogenic properties of many commercial sun protection products.

To understand how to sift through these contradictory messages, it is important to realize that what you read in the headlines or hear in media sound bites is often too simplistic. Take, for instance, the suggestion that if you spend "fifteen minutes a day" in the sun, three times per week, that will ensure that the body will produce sufficient vitamin D. As you already know from developing sun sense (in Chapter 2), you won't be able to produce any D at all unless you're exposed to UVB rays—and those rays are only available at certain times of day, year, and in certain latitudes. On a summer day, the intensity of UVBs in Canada will be less than the intensity of those rays on a Florida beach in the United States. In addition, your skin type will alert you that if you burn easily, that recommended "fifteen minutes a day" could result in sunburn, depending on the intensity of the UVB rays.

When it comes to sun exposure, the "one-size-fits-all" advice simply does not work for the six billion individuals on the planet. Interestingly, since I have developed sun sense, I find that I protect my skin , especially my head and face, throughout the day and consciously expose my skin in the right circumstances. In order to protect your skin, it's helpful if you think of your time in the sun as divided into two distinct segments:

- sensible sun exposure for vitamin D
- everyday sun exposure

We will take a look at both of these options in the next section.

Steps to Sensible Sun Exposure for Vitamin D

Before you attempt to sunbathe or expose your skin to the sun to begin producing vitamin D, you will need to gather basic information and follow these steps:

1. Determine your skin type: As explained in Chapter 3, your propensity to tan or burn depends upon your skin type. Your skin type also affects how long you need to stay in the sun to trigger the process of creating vitamin D—and how much or how little sun you can get before burning. Remember: Never burn your skin.

   CAUTION: Depending on certain health issues and the severity of the condition, it is questionable whether any sun exposure is appropriate for some people. Consult with your dermatologist or other health-care provider before you expose your skin to the sun if you are sun sensitive or HIV positive, if you have lupus, if you are taking medications, or if you have other conditions where sun exposure is contraindicated.

2. Know your MED: Your personal MED, which, again, stands for "minimal erythemal dose," is the longest amount of time you can spend in the sun before running the risk of having your skin turn red twenty-four hours after exposure. Depending on your skin type, the season of the year, the time of day, the latitude, etc., that dose may be only a few minutes; it also may be a half hour. If you recall from Chapter 3, knowing your MED is not a precise science. Rather, it is a matter of paying attention to your body and knowing how it responds to the sun.

3. Verify UV Index: The best way to access the UV Index in your area is through websites for up-to-date reports, weather stations online, or apps for your phone. You can purchase a hand-held UVB monitor that some people find helpful.

4. Start slowly: Go for the smallest dose of sun exposure that you are confident will not cause sunburn. If your personal MED is twenty minutes when the UV Index is 6, then stay out for only five or six minutes during the first session. Then gradually increase the time by one to three minutes each session—but stop when you reach 50 percent of your MED.

    CAUTION: Dark skin can burn, too, particularly in body areas that are not ordinarily exposed. Therefore, both dark- and light-skinned people should always begin a sunbathing regimen slowly.

5. Expose the best skin areas: To reap the benefits of sensible sunbathing, you will want to let the sun's UVB rays touch as much of your body as you can. That means you will not be using sunscreen. But do cover body areas that have had significant lifetime exposure, such as the face, your shoulders, and

the tops of your ears and arms. Give more time to the inner arms and other areas that have only had minimal previous exposure to the sun.

6. Repeat this process: Repeat this type of sun exposure two to three times per week when conditions are right, and your body will begin to produce healthy amounts of vitamin D. (But keep in mind—it is highly unlikely that you will be able to make enough D from the sun alone, so you still will need to take supplements as well, especially if you live at a latitude above or below 37°—see Chapter 2.)

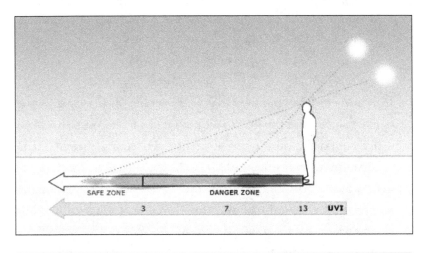

Exposure Category	Index Number	Sun-Protection Messages
LOW	<2	You can safely be outdoors with minimal protection. If you burn easily, use sunscreen.
MODERATE	3 to 5	Sun exposure can cause damage. Take precautions, such as covering up. Stay in shade near midday when the sun is strongest. Use SPF 30+ every two hours.

Exposure Category	Index Number	Sun-Protection Messages
HIGH	6 to 7	High risk of harm. Protection against sunburn is needed. Cover up; wear a hat and sunglasses. Reduce time in the sun between 10 a.m. and 4 p.m. Use SPF 30+.
VERY HIGH	8 to 10	Very high risk. Take extra precautions. Unprotected skin will be damaged and can burn quickly. Seek shade, cover up, and wear a hat and sunglasses. Avoid sun between 10 a.m. and 4 p.m. Use SPF 30+.
EXTREME	11+	Extreme danger. Take ALL precautions. Unprotected skin can burn in minutes. Seek shade, cover up, and wear a hat and sunglasses. Avoid the sun between 10 a.m. and 4 p.m. Use SPF 30+.

UV Index Chart for UVB Rays Only (Figure 11.2)

The UV Index only pertains to UVB rays. Remember, UVA rays are strong *all day long* and highest at solar noon, and can result in skin damage, but not sunburn, which is why daily sun-protection strategies are important throughout the day, as you can read about it in Chapter 2. Hats are strongly recommend throughout the day to protect from both UVB and UVA damage.

Why Would Anyone Who Has Had Skin Cancer Sunbathe?

While I have had many skin cancers due to my early-in-life second-degree sunburns, I do expose some of my skin for vitamin D production and other benefits that I believe I get when I sunbathe. I live above latitude 37° in the San Francisco Bay area, so in the winter vitamin D–producing UVB rays are scarce. Also, during the summer we have UVB blocking fog. Understanding the sun and atmospheric conditions has allowed me to have a safe relationship with the sun while reaping the benefits. The following is an example of how I interact with the sun mindfully for sunbathing.

I always check the UV Index to determine the best time for me to expose my type 3 skin. I avoid a UV Index above 6. My MED for a UV Index of 6 is twenty minutes. I stay out no longer than ten minutes on each side of my body. My face is completely covered with dark and thick material. I never develop the slightest redness. Over time I do develop a very light tan, which while not recommended by most dermatologists, I feel comfortable with it.

Vitamin D (UVB) Lamps—Yes or No?

If you are unable to sunbathe for vitamin D in the sun, should you consider purchasing a UVB lamp or go to a tanning salon? In this section, we will look at UVB lamps for home use.

When our bodies are exposed to UVB rays, the skin produces at least six different substances, including vitamin D. We are learning about the added benefits of these substances, discussed in Chapter 4. As we learn more about these substances, we may find that they provide additional health benefits.

So if you live in a sun-deprived area or you are unable to absorb vitamin D, should you consider a UVB lamp? For some people with health issues such as malabsorption problems, surgical removal of small intestines, etc., skin production of vitamin D would be desirable. Also, some skin conditions are treated with UV lamp radiation, including psoriasis. For most of us, getting some of our vitamin D can be obtained safely through sensible sun exposure, and that method may be more beneficial than taking supplements, especially because of the other substances formed from exposure to UVB rays.

So, if you live in a latitude above or below 37°, or in an area with tall buildings, chronic fog, or in any other situation that limits your skin's ability to produce vitamin D, perhaps a home unit is a good option for you. Among the lamps available for purchase, you will find those that emit UVB with a small amount of UVA. The advantage of a home unit versus a tanning salon unit is that you will know exactly what kind of bulb is used, and remember, salons for tanning increase the dose of UVA rays to dangerous levels.

There are vitamin D lightboxes that you can purchase. One company that I have tried, the Sperti lamp, increases or maintains D levels. As a disclaimer, I have no commercial connection with this company.

Note:

Questioning the Research of Sunbed Tanning by Michael Holick, MD

Researcher Michael Holick has come under scrutiny for monetarily benefiting from the sunbed industry and vitamin D testing. It has been reported that he has been paid by the sunbed industry for supporting the use of sunbeds for the purpose of producing vitamin D. He has also been accused of benefiting from vitamin D testing sales.

Michael Holick's research stands on its own and his findings provide consumers with very important information regarding vitamin D deficiency and health issues. However, I do not recommend the use of sun-tanning salons because that tan comes at a cost. Most facilities, in order to get you out the door more quickly, use a high dose of UVA—7 to 10 times what the sun emits. You will remember from earlier chapters that UVA rays are the rays that tan our skin. That said, they also penetrate deeply within the skin layers, and can result in future skin cancers.

To minimize skin damage and the risk of skin cancer, carefully follow the lamp's instructions, and make sure you use your equipment according to your skin type and MED and expose body areas that have had the least sun exposure, such as your inner arms and other areas that are typically covered with clothing.

Everyday Sun Exposure

Besides deliberately engaging in limited sun exposure sessions to produce vitamin D, you also need to develop a healthy relationship with the sun in your *everyday* life. It is important to be aware of the consequences of everyday cumulative sun exposure.

Here are a few tips on staying safe in the sun every day:

- Skin protection must become a daily habit of choosing protective clothing, wearing hats, and applying sunscreen products that are safe. (You will learn about these in Chapter 12.)
- Remember: When you squint, that's a hint! Squinting is a clue that the sunlight may be too bright for your eyes. Use good-quality sunglasses in extremely bright sunlight. The best color for sunglasses is gray, as it does not distort light as much as other colors.
- Avoid the midday sun as much as possible. To play it safe, especially on vacation, plan sun activities earlier or later in the day.
- Use non-chemical sunscreen (see Chapter 12) and reapply it periodically when engaging in active sports or swimming. And that may mean reapplying it hourly!
- UVA rays, which both tan and age the skin, can penetrate window glass. While it may feel good to sit next to a warm window (as many cats and dogs demonstrate), you should be aware of the potential for cumulative sun damage. Remember

too: UVB rays cannot penetrate glass, so you will not make vitamin D when sitting near a sunny window.

■ As when sunbathing for vitamin D, your daily sun exposure should also consider the need to cover up and protect areas of your body that have received significant exposure during the course of your lifetime—the face, shoulders, ears, and particularly, the nose. Legs for many women (especially back of legs) and men's backs or the tops of their heads have often received significant lifetime sun exposure. Having several sun hats to choose from in your home and car should make it easy for you to keep these areas protected.

Get to Know Your Shadow Side: Sensible Sun Protection Strategies

Now that you've gotten a good overview on the best ways to handle everyday sun exposure, let's take a more detailed look at the best commonsense strategies for protecting your skin from excess UV radiation.

We'll begin with a typical scenario: Suppose you're getting ready for the beach or a barbecue. You might grab a straw hat and a pair of lightly-tinted sunglasses to prepare for a day outdoors. Perhaps you bring along a faded beach umbrella for shade, and some families pack white T-shirts to cover up the kids when they go swimming. Like many people, you probably assume these items will protect you from UV radiation. Unfortunately, that assumption is wrong. Here's why:

■ Loosely woven straw hats allow UVA and UVB rays to pass right through them and hit your skin directly.

■ Sunglasses without dark lenses and full-spectrum protection do little to prevent damage to your eyes.

■ Even if a faded, pale beach umbrella provides some shade, it does not really block out much of the UV radiation. Many people end up with severe sunburns at the end of the day despite being under an umbrella.

■ T-shirts, especially white, do not fully prevent penetration of the sun's rays, and offer even less protection once they become wet and stretched, which typically happens when they're worn by swimmers.

The real problem with any of these measures is that people believe they are doing the right thing—such as wearing a hat or sunglasses— to take care of themselves. They therefore develop a false sense of security and don't pursue the types of sunburn prevention efforts that are, in fact, effective.

What can you do to stop wasting time and money on methods and products that don't actually keep your skin safe? Knowing which types of garments and textiles to look for is one good place to start, since clothes provide some of the best protection available, and that's what you'll learn about next.

Sensible Sunwear

Part of developing sun sense is to recognize that you need to be prepared with the proper types of garments to protect your skin from excess UV radiation. No one would think twice about carrying an umbrella when it looks like rain, but most of us are not as conscious about keeping sun protection gear on hand. The tips below will give you guidelines about the type of clothing and accessories you need— but you'll have to make the effort to put these items in your car or place them near your front door so that you'll make real use of them.

Protective Clothing Tips

Keep these points in mind when buying or selecting clothes for sunburn prevention purposes:

Tight Weave: The weave of a fabric is the most important factor in terms of UV protection. A fabric with a loose weave (such as lace or a very lightweight material) allows light to pass through it and is not as protective as cloth that is tightly woven, such as bamboo, Lycra, or even polyester. You can check the weave of a fabric by holding it up to a window to see how much light shines through. Although this test is not perfect, it can give you an idea.

Color: Besides having a tight weave, color is the next most important determinant of a fabric's ability to protect your skin from excess exposure to UV rays. Dark colors—including browns, blacks, and grays as well as blues, greens, and reds—tend to absorb UV radiation, so they offer better protection than white or light-colored fabrics, which allow UV rays to go through them. Because dark-colored clothes absorb light, they can create more body heat; so, if you are extremely active on hot summer days, you may want to search out specially designed sportswear that provides sun protection while also keeping you cool.

Thickness/Stretch: The thicker the fabric, the more UV rays it can absorb, and conversely, the thinner the fabric, the less it absorbs. Further, when a fabric is stretched, its "thickness" diminishes and UV rays can slip past the spaces between the threads, which means that stretchy fabrics are less effective as sun cover-ups.

Wetness: When fabric gets wet, UV rays penetrate it more easily. That is why you (or your children) should not rely on a white or faded T-shirt to protect your skin when swimming.

Hats, Caps, and Visors: Hats with thick, wide brims are the most protective. Typically, straw hats are so loosely woven that they allow UV rays to penetrate through them. Manufacturers are beginning to market tightly-woven straw hats for sun protection; but, as with fabric, you should double-check these headpieces by holding them up to the sunlight to see if any rays get through.

Caps with a thick brim may shade your face from the sun. But generally, baseball caps (or other styles of caps) *do not* fully protect you, especially because they leave your ears and the back of your neck exposed.

Visors also do not protect the ears or the back of the neck, and they leave the top of your head exposed, making it more susceptible to skin damage. In recent years, "full face" or "extra-long" visors have gained in popularity in countries like Japan, and these types of head coverings do offer more protection than traditional visors. But some styles of full-face visors can make wearers look like Darth Vader from the Star Wars movies, so they have not caught on everywhere.

Swimwear: In Australia, where skin cancer is very common, it is also common to see people wearing swimwear that covers a significant portion of the body. This type of swimwear is particularly appropriate for regular swimmers whose lifetime sun exposure is high. For maximum sun protection, look for styles with high collars, sleeves, and longer pant legs in darker-colored fabrics.

Umbrellas: Many beach umbrellas are lightweight and light-colored. They offer little defense against UV radiation, and people can get sunburned sitting under them. As with other types of sun protection fabric, look for umbrellas that are tightly woven and dark colored. Basically, very little, if any light should pass through an umbrella. Besides large beach umbrellas, smaller umbrellas have traditionally provided cooling shade for people walking around under the tropical sun. These "sun umbrellas" and old-fashioned parasols are also beginning to appear in more northern climates as well, as people become more conscious about protecting their skin from excess sun.

My Personal Sun Protection Strategies

Because of my personal experience with skin cancer and my commitment to a conscious relationship with the sun, I make it a habit to put on a wide-brimmed hat with solid material that prevents UV penetration. Hats, I believe, are a must, even when going to or from the car or mailbox, but the hat fabric must be tightly woven or else UV rays can pass through the material, which defeats the whole purpose of the hat.

Walking around without shading your face in the early morning or late afternoon will not increase vitamin D, and it exposes you unnecessarily to UVA rays and skin damage. (Remember, you can only produce vitamin D when UVB rays interact with your skin, and you also need to follow the other "sensible sunbathing" tips given in Chapter 4.

Besides having easy access to a variety of hats (either hanging near my front door or stashed in my car), I also carry a sarong, which is a long piece of material from Bali that is three feet long and 30 inches wide. It can cover my legs or shoulders when I'm in the sun. I keep bandanas around for the same purpose and also use them in my car window when I'm stuck in traffic. (I simply roll down the side window, and put the edge of a bandana on the top of the glass, and roll it back up to keep it in place.)

Ultraviolet Protection Factor (UPF) for Clothing

The UPF rating is a relatively new rating for sun protective textiles and clothing, which represents the ratio of sunburn-causing UV measured without and with the protection of the fabric.

Like SPF, the higher the number, the less UV radiation that passes through. A fabric rated UPF 15 allows 7 percent of UVB rays that burn to pass through. UPF 50 allows 2 percent of UVB rays to pass.

The UPF number does not convey the effectiveness of UVA protection. This is usually not a problem because protection offered by clothing is naturally well balanced between UVA and UVB. A shirt that blocks most UVB rays will also block most UVA rays. In contrast, a high SPF sunscreen may filter UVB rays well, but that's no guarantee of good UVA protection.

Besides having a tight weave or dark color, clothing today also can be "UPF-rated" or marketed as being made from "sun protection fabric"; it might also be "chemically treated" to absorb UV radiation. I must admit that the first time I saw a tag hanging from a shirt with a UPF rating, I rolled my eyes and thought to myself, "Yet another sales gimmick using fear tactics to market things to people!" Upon further investigation, however, I began to feel that these garments might have an appropriate use. I'm not entirely convinced that the average person needs them for most activities—after all, wearing a plain dark-colored, long-sleeved shirt can usually protect you just fine. But, particularly for athletes and other active people, as well as for those people who are very sun sensitive or who work outdoors most of the time, it might be worthwhile to wear clothing that has built-in sun protection.

As with understanding how chemical and mineral sunscreens work (as explained in Chapter 12), you will have to wade through a variety of labels and marketing claims to figure out how sun-protective clothing could meet your needs. The following overview of some basic terms and concepts should help you cut through the hype about these types of garments.

SPF and UPF—What's the Difference?

While you may be familiar with the SPF ratings on sunscreen bottles, you probably know less about the UPF ratings on clothes. The box below captures how these terms differ.

SPF	UPF
stands for "sun protection factor"	stands for "ultraviolet protection factor"
rates sunscreens	rates clothing and textiles
estimates the amount of time it takes for a person's unprotected skin to burn	measures how much ultraviolet radiation penetrates a fabric and reaches the skin
refers *only* to the degree of protection against UVB rays	refers to the amount of protection a fabric offers against both UVB and UVA rays
is regulated in the United States by the Food and Drug Administration (FDA)	Federal Trade Commission regulates these products by overseeing marketing advertising claims.

Different countries, different labeling

In Europe and Australia their labeling system is different, and frankly better, than the United States. They do use the SPF rating as we do in the United States; however, they also use a star system.

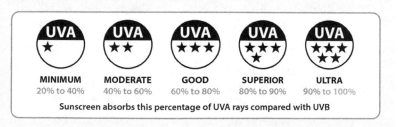

MINIMUM 20% to 40%   MODERATE 40% to 60%   GOOD 60% to 80%   SUPERIOR 80% to 90%   ULTRA 90% to 100%

Sunscreen absorbs this percentage of UVA rays compared with UVB

UVA Star Rating System: In the UK and Ireland, the Boots star rating system is a proprietary in vitro method used to describe the ratio of UVA to UVB protection offered by sunscreen products.

The stars range from 0 to 5 and indicate the percentage of UVA radiation absorbed by the sunscreen in comparison to UVB, in other words the ratio between the level of protection afforded by the UVA protection and the UVB protection.

Be aware that if you choose a low SPF it may still have a high level of stars, not because it is providing lots of UVA protection, but because the ratio between the UVA and UVB protection is about the same.

It's important to choose a high SPF as well as a high UVA protection (high number of stars). Sunscreens that offer both UVA and UVB protection are sometimes called "broad spectrum." A sunscreen with an SPF of 30 and a UVA rating of 4 or 5 stars is generally considered as a good standard of sun protection in addition to shade and clothing.

UPF Ratings: What Do They Mean?

To understand UPF ratings for "sun-protection fabrics," it's helpful to know how garments with different ratings compare. For example, the plain white T-shirt often seen at the beach may have a UPF of only 5 or 6, but a pair of dark-brown pants made from thick corduroy would likely get a UPF rating of about 50. A fabric with a rating of 50 will allow only 1/50 of the sun's UV rays to pass through. This reduces your skin's UV radiation exposure by 1 percent; only 3 percent of the UV rays will penetrate to the skin covered by a UPF 50-rated garment.

The effectiveness of a garment's UPF rating is ranked according to the table below, which shows the guidelines established by the Australian/New Zealand standards for sun-protective clothing and swimwear (considered the industry standard for sun-protective clothing).

UPF RATINGS

UPF Rating	Protection Category	% of UV Radiation Blocked
UPF 15 to 24	Good	93.3 to 95.9
UPF 25 to 39	Very Good	96.0 to 97.4
UPF 40 to 50+	Excellent	97.5 to 98+

Chemically Treated Clothing: Buyer Beware

Just as chemical sunscreens can absorb UV radiation to prevent sunburn, so can fabrics also be chemically treated to absorb these rays, and some companies use this type of treatment in their sun-protective clothing lines. Since I am always concerned about the excess use of chemicals, I prefer products and clothing that do not add unnecessary chemicals. Because the whole field of sun-protective clothing is evolving, you will have to carefully check labels and company websites to determine how a piece of clothing achieves its UPF rating: through the tight weave or through chemicals. One method of creating UV-blocking clothes is to weave titanium dioxide into the fabric. Given that titanium has proven safe for years, I would opt for companies using this naturally occurring mineral.

Other problems that arise with chemically treated sun-protection fabrics are that the clothes lose their effectiveness after numerous washings and the chemicals end up in our water supply. Clothing manufacturers are working to create products that will withstand the laundry process. Taking a different approach to the issue, the RIT company, long-known for producing fabric dyes, offers a product called SunGuard™ that enables you to add UV-blocking protection to clothes when washing them at home. The product label states that it has the protection equivalent of SPF 30, which lasts through twenty washings. It remains to be seen what long-term effects these chemicals will have on our environment in the future since it ends up in water, including water from washing garments, and the waters in which we swim. We do know, through studies, that fish swimming in water with endocrine disrupting chemicals exhibit signs of hormone disruption. You will learn more about this in chapter 12.

The following excerpt is from the Environmental Working Group website regarding UPF-rated fabrics and the substances that are used in the fabric to achieve a UPF rating for UV rays.

"Over the past two decades, clothing claiming an ultraviolet protection factor—UPF for short—has enjoyed a soaring growth curve. A recent search of the Amazon website for sun protective clothing returned nearly 25,000 products.

"UPF clothing is distinguished from regular clothes by lab tests that show it shields the body from UV rays by a factor of 15 or greater. For everyday use, most clothing without a UPF label can provide adequate sun protection. A white cotton shirt's UPF may hover around 10. A colored shirt's UPF is higher. Denim jeans can have a UPF value of 1700. The reason: tighter weaves, dark or bright colors and thicker fabrics block more UV rays. If the fabric is wet, stretched out or too tight, it will block fewer UV rays. Some additives such as minerals including titanium dioxide, zinc oxide and Tinosorb FD are infused into fabric to improve UV filtering, but I don't advise buying clothes infused with chemicals."

Fabrics Treated with Chemicals to Repel Mosquitoes, Ticks, and Biting Insects?

No discussion of chemically treated fabric is complete without mentioning apparel made of cloth infused with insect-repelling chemicals. The repellent is supposed to last for twenty to thirty washings. I do not recommend the use of these garments. If someone does choose to buy them, they should use them sparingly and only when it is absolutely necessary. The chemicals that make these garments are effective as insect repellents, but they are also toxic, and they eventually end up in the environment. Even more disturbing is that in DEET is a known endocrine disruptor.

DEET is not only a fabric additive, it is also the repellent ingredient in some products that are made to be applied directly to the skin. I definitely do not recommend applying DEET to the skin, if at all possible. If you feel you have no choice but to use a DEET-containing insect repellent, buy a product that has a stick applicator, and apply it to pant cuffs, shoes, socks, and shirt collars. Another effective way to use DEET is to apply some to a bandana that you can tie around your neck, and dot some on clothing. In my experience, some repellents that do not contain DEET, though less effective in general, are effective enough when not inundated with mosquitoes.

Remember, sprays of *any* kind pose additional health hazards because the chemicals they contain can be inhaled and damage the lungs. Natural bug repellents—such as citronella oil, cinnamon, lemon eucalyptus, orange oil, and rose geranium—can also be effective. Apply caution with natural products, too, however, as they can be dangerous if children (or others) ingest them; some people have allergic reactions to some of these substances as well.

Chapter Wrap-up: Simple Sun-Protection Strategies

Following is a recap of the various ways you can keep your skin from getting burned by the sun

Wear hats: Buy several wide-brimmed, tightly woven hats and keep a stock of them in your car and near the front door. Make a habit of wearing hats when going outside—especially for sun-intense situations.

Wear bandanas/scarves: Scarves and bandanas can serve as emergency protection. They can be worn with a baseball cap and hung down over the back of the neck (to protect both your neck and your ears), or they can be used to cover an exposed limb.

Choose tight-weave garments: Whether a piece of clothing has a UPF (ultraviolet protection factor) rating or not, make sure it is a tight-weave to block harmful rays.

Color matters: The darker the garment, the more protection it offers. Gray, dark blue, and black are the best UV absorbers.

Choose long-sleeved shirts and pants: Covering your arms and legs with long-sleeved shirts and long pants will help prevent UV radiation from reaching your skin—if the fabric is tightly woven.

Drink water: Well-hydrated skin is more resilient. It is important to rehydrate for fluids lost to sweating.

Wear sunglasses: Wear full-spectrum sunglasses for both UVA and UVB protection. Be sure the sunglasses you choose are rated full spectrum 100 percent protection. Have an optometrist check your sunglasses for UV protection, since many of them do not live up to claims advertised on the label.

Don't count on beach umbrellas: Most inexpensive beach umbrellas are not tightly woven or dark enough to provide full UV protection. You can still get a sunburn sitting under a lightweight umbrella.

Be aware of ground surfaces: Sand, cement, and white-painted surfaces—as well as the snow—reflect the sun's rays. In water, UV light penetrates to three-feet deep.

Stay sun aware in cars: Use a bandana to cover your arm when you are driving or to block the sun from hitting a child's face in the back seat—or use roll-down window shades on car windows for that purpose.

Practice the "shadow rule": Look for shade when your shadow is shorter than you are tall.

Use chemical-free sunscreens: Look for titanium dioxide or zinc in sunscreens, which are the best choice. If you must use chemicals in sunscreens, choose the ones that are rated safe and are not known carcinogens. (See Chapter 12 for details.)

Shining Light on . . . Children and the Sun

Just as "sensible sunbathing" can be useful for adults to produce vitamin D through consciously and strategically exposing themselves to the sun, so, too, can most children benefit from being out in the daylight. Controlled sun exposure is good for children. But it is good only if parents and caregivers protect children from excess sun exposure with the same vigilance and consistency as they use in protecting them from extreme cold and rain.

Making sure our kids wear all the gear—hats, boots, jackets, mittens, mufflers—appropriate for cold or rain is second nature. But when it comes to sun protection, it's not so easy because the most sun-intense and dangerous times are just the times when kids are most likely to want to shed their restrictive clothes and be outdoors. Skin damage is cumulative and starts with that first, seemingly innocent sunburn. Even one serious sunburn before age eighteen can significantly increase the risk of developing skin cancers later in life.

With the specter of possible future skin cancer in mind, you may well ask, "Do children need to use sunscreen every day?" If a child has light skin, burns easily, and lives in a sun-intense area, the answer is yes. For these children, use all protection avenues: limit the amount of time in the sun, dress them in protective clothing, and use sunscreen on skin areas not covered by clothing. Children with blond, red, or light-brown hair and blue, green, or gray eyes need close monitoring and extra precautions, and so do children with a lot of moles.

It is important to balance our concerns for children's sensitive skin with the equally important need to ensure that some of their vitamin D is obtained through sensible sun exposure. Remember: sunscreens with an SPF 30 rating reduces vitamin D production by approximately 97 percent.

One further complication for today's parent is that more young children are spending a significant amount of their daylight hours at daycare centers, where they (and their parents) depend upon the caregivers to manage sun protection as well as to ensure that the kids get regular playtime in the sun. Make sure your child's daycare program includes daily outdoor time and that the staff is educated and diligent about sun protection for all the children in their care. In schools and daycare centers most facilities use spray sunscreens that are chemically based. If you want your child to use a better product you will likely need to supply it.

On weekends and vacations, parents need to think through their children's activities to make sure that both they and their children are equipped with what they will need for sun protection before leaving for extended trips or activities with long hours of potential sun exposure.

Protection for Infants and Children

So, what can we do to help our kids enjoy the outdoors while protecting them from sun damage? Here are a few of the things that should become standard operating procedure in households with children:

- Provide sun-protective clothing such as long pants and long sleeves.
- Avoid midday sun as much as possible and plan sun activities early or late in the day, and limit the amount of time in the sun.
- Find shade: Check to see how shaded the play areas are and direct activities to the shaded area when possible.
- Apply sunscreen on your child before he or she leaves the house; apply a non-chemical sun protection factor (SPF) of at least 30 to block the most harmful sunrays. Don't forget the lips, backs of hands, and feet. Zinc is the safest and most protective active ingredient for everyone, including children.
- Reapply sunscreen every hour when necessary. Teach children how to use sunscreen and to reapply it when appropriate (such as during intense sun exposure or when protection wears off from sweating or swimming).
- Keep infants out of direct sun altogether and covered up— never apply sunscreen to children under six months old. This is clearly the safest recommendation as not all parents are fully present.
- Shade car windows: Shade your children from the sun's rays if they are sitting near a window. No vitamin D–producing rays (UVB) penetrate glass. UVA rays, which cause skin damage, do pass through glass, so I think press-on or pulldown shades are worthwhile. They can be purchased in automotive stores or online. As I note, adults should have these shades

available, too, for when the sun is shining directly through the side windows.

As we have learned, we should be thinking about protecting our skin from damaging sunrays every day, even if it is cloudy or foggy. We have also learned that complete sun avoidance is not healthy and that there is a middle ground between protecting and interacting with the sun consciously. As we move forward with understanding how to minimize skin damage from the sun, the number one thing to remember is to avoid chronic, excessive sun exposure on the skin and don't get burned!

Key Points from Chapter 11 — Sensible Sun Exposure and Sun Protection

- Know your MED

- Sensible sun-exposure is mindful sun-exposure

- Always carry hats and other clothing in your car to protect you and your family

- If you avoid the sun, check your vitamin D level and calcium too

- Check the UV Index in your area—weather channels show the index daily

- Sunbeds are not recommended—they increase UVA rays 7–15 times what the sun emits

Chapter 12

Safe Sunscreens and Chemicals to Avoid

If sunburns contribute to skin cancer, then it makes sense to stop those burns by using sunscreen, right?

Not exactly.

Yes, when used properly, sunscreen products along with commonsense measures can prevent sunburns and skin damage. But I have concerns regarding some of the chemicals used in sunscreen products. The chemicals in many commercial sunscreens have been linked to hormonal activity, allergies, and even carcinogenic DNA damage. On top of that, sunscreens are often misused, and their labeling can be misleading.

Because many people do not stop to consider these issues before they rub these products all over their bodies, this chapter will examine the various problems posed by sunscreen use, and where possible, it will also offer solutions.

Today the term *sunscreen* includes both chemical and mineral active ingredients. Mineral sunscreen used to be called sunblock. In 2011, the FDA passed new regulations regarding product labeling that prohibited companies from identifying a product as a sunblock. They did this because there was a lot of confusion for consumers. Zinc and titanium are minerals that, prior to the new regulation, were referred to as sunblock because they stay on top of the skin providing a *physical block* reflecting the sun's rays. While I liked the term *sunblock,* because minerals do work very differently than chemicals, I basically agree with the change. Now consumers understand what they are buying and read labels.

While there is a lot of information to digest, rest assured, you will be able to select the safest products for you and your family. Now let's take a deep dive into sunscreen ingredients.

Mineral vs. Chemical Sunscreens— How Do They Work?

People are still confused, and you will continue to see the words *sunscreen* and *sunblock* used interchangeably in news stories and websites, but these two approaches to protecting your skin from the effects of harmful ultraviolet (UV) radiation are not identical. Consider the following explanations as we take a closer look at how each of these skin protection methods work.

- Chemical sunscreens: the type that most people purchase at drug stores and use for the beach and other outdoor activities. They mostly contain chemicals that soak into your skin and create a protective layer that absorbs UV rays and disperses them as heat. In order to prevent the "full spectrum" of UV light from damaging the skin, sunscreens need at least one chemical for absorbing UVB rays and one (or more) separate chemicals for UVA rays, which means that the formulations for these sunscreen products usually contain multiple chemicals and the product label may read, "broad spectrum."

- Mineral sunscreens: contain minerals, such as titanium dioxide or zinc oxide, which do not penetrate the skin and are not absorbed into it. Rather, these minerals sit on top of the skin and block or reflect the sun's rays like thousands of tiny mirrors, scattering the ultraviolet radiation. Minerals provide protection for both UVB and UVA rays, and therefore they can include "broad spectrum" on their labels.

Label Requirements for Sunscreens

The following is an excerpt of new labeling requirements for sunscreens from the U.S. Food and Drug Administration website:

- Broad-spectrum designation. Sunscreens that pass the FDA's broad-spectrum test procedure, which measures a product's UVB and UVA protection, may be labeled as "Broad Spectrum SPF" on the front label. For broad-spectrum sunscreens, SPF values also indicate the amount or magnitude of overall protection. Broad-spectrum SPF products with SPF values higher than 15 provide greater protection and may claim additional uses, as described in the next bullet.

- Use claims. Only broad-spectrum sunscreens with an SPF value of 15 or higher can claim to reduce the risk of skin cancer and early skin aging, if used as directed, with other sun protection measures. Sunscreens with an SPF between 2 and 14 can claim only to help prevent sunburn.

- "Waterproof," "sweatproof," or "sunscreen" claims. Manufacturers cannot label sunscreens as "waterproof" or "sweatproof" because these claims overstate their effectiveness. Sunscreens also cannot claim to provide sun protection for more than two hours without reapplication or to provide protection immediately after application (for example, "instant protection") without submitting data to support these claims and obtaining FDA approval.

- Water-resistance claims. Water-resistance claims on the front label must indicate whether the sunscreen remains effective for forty minutes or eighty minutes while swimming or sweating, based on standard testing. Sunscreens that are not water resistant must include a direction instructing consumers to use a water-resistant sunscreen if swimming or sweating.

Now that we understand the claims that can be made, let's look at the ingredient lists that are typically on the back of these products. Below you will learn about two lists: active and inactive ingredients.

Active Ingredients

Active ingredients, as the name suggests, are those parts of a formulation that directly activate a product and create the effect the product is designed to achieve. Everything listed in active ingredients is either a chemical or a mineral.

Inactive Ingredients in Sunscreen Products—What Should You Look For?

Inactive ingredients, sometimes called "inert ingredients," do not directly produce a certain effect, but they may improve the stability, appearance, or usability of a product, among other things. The inactive ingredients list includes the base ingredients, such as oils, blending agents, fragrance, and preservatives, and many of these pose health risks that will be detailed later in this chapter.

Remember, as discussed earlier in this book, the skin is your largest organ and what you put on the outside of your body can often be absorbed into your bloodstream. Since sunscreens are typically lotions, you will find that many have the same ingredients as your face and body moisturizers.

For now, just remember that when you evaluate a product, you need to examine the list of both active and inactive ingredients before purchasing it.

Making Sense of SPFs

Sunscreens are rated and labeled with a sun protection factor (SPF) that measures the fraction of sunburn-producing UVB rays that reach the skin. For example, "SPF 15" means that $\frac{1}{15}$ of the burning radiation reaches the skin through the recommended thickness of sunscreen. Another way to understand this is that an SPF of 15 will supposedly allow you to be out in the sun fifteen times longer without burning than without it. Keep in mind this varies with skin type and whether or not you slap on enough of the product to provide the protection that is listed.

SPF rating pertains only to UVB rays. That is because UVB rays are responsible for burning the skin, and when the rating system was first implemented, UVA rays were generally thought to be safe. In recent years, UVA rays have been associated with multiple forms of skin cancer and deep wrinkling of the skin. Early chemical sunscreen products only screened UVB rays, which allowed the UVA rays to penetrate the skin of sunscreen users, for hours on end in some cases. As noted in Chapter 9, this lack of protection against UVA rays is one of the factors contributing to the increase in skin-cancer rates over the past couple of decades.

Now that we understand the abbreviation "SPF," keep in mind that it *only* pertains to UVB rays. The term "broad-spectrum" pertains to both UVB and UVA. To make the best use of information about SPFs in a product, it helps to know some additional information:

- If you recall from Chapter 3, your MED stands for minimal erythemal dose, that is the amount of sunlight that will cause your unprotected skin to redden or turn pink within twenty-four hours after sun exposure.
- The SPF of a product considers the amount of time it takes for a person's protected skin to redden (or reach its MED), compared to the amount of time needed for that person's unprotected skin. This means that if the skin turns pink within twenty-four hours of being in the sun—this is MED—you can safely stay out in the sun half that time.

■ The SPF protection is only met if the product is applied correctly—meaning a thick coat. As an example, if an SPF 15 is applied thinly the protection value may only be an SPF 8.

When applied correctly, an SPF 30 will afford you the protection of one minute of UVB rays for each thirty minutes you spend in the sun. So, one hour in the sun wearing SPF 30 sunscreen is the same as spending two minutes totally unprotected.

Understanding SPF Protection: Although the FDA has proposed regulations to prevent companies from labeling their products as having an SPF higher than SPF 50+, that has not stopped all manufacturers from making such claims. A sunscreen with SPF value in the range of 30 to 50 will offer adequate sunburn protection against UVB rays for most people. When *initially* applied, sunscreens offer the following protection—assuming proper application, perfect weather conditions, and reasonable UV intensity:

SPF 15 = 93 percent

SPF 30 = 97 percent

SPF 40 = 97.5 percent

SPF 50 = 98 percent

SPF 100+ = 99 percent

High SPF products require higher concentrations of sun-filtering chemicals than lower SPF sunscreens. Basically, a high SPF, over 50, only offers an additional one percent protection and exposes you to more chemicals that you do not need.

Active Ingredients to Use and Avoid

Active ingredients apply to UVB and UVA rays. As covered above, there is no SPF rating for UVA—only a product that states "broad spectrum" can make that claim.

Hands down, zinc oxide is the most effective broad-spectrum active ingredient. It is the *only* active ingredient that I feel comfortable recommending. It is safer and more effective at blocking both UVA and UVB.

Chemicals target either UVB rays or UVA rays. This is why multiple chemicals are needed to provide a full-spectrum rating.

The toxicity of some of the active ingredients is of great concern for humans, animals, and even coral reefs. Many of the chemicals have been shown to disrupt hormonal activity as you will see in the chart below. Recall again that the skin is our largest organ, and it is permeable to many of the substances we put on it. That is why medications, including hormones and nicotine patches, can be delivered via "transdermal" (through the skin) applications.

See the chart below regarding the most common active ingredients. There are *many* more ingredients, some approved in the United States, Japan and Australia, many of which are concerning and are banned in certain countries. Also, there are many more chemicals that are approved for use in the United States that are not on this chart. You can view an ongoing list at Wikipedia under Sunscreens. The following list is adapted from the 2018 Environmental Working Group website. (For updates, visit EWG.org.) Most of these active ingredients are common in the United States and have been rated by EWG. Any of the names for the chemicals can be found on sunscreen labels.

Chemical or Mineral	EWG Hazard Score	Use in U.S. Sunscreens and filter type	Skin Penetration	Hormone disruption	Skin Allergy	Other Concerns
Oxybenzone Benzophenone-3, Eusolex 4360, Escalol 567 *Banned in Hawaii*	8 UVB only	Widespread	Detected in nearly every American; found in mothers' milk; 1% to 9% skin penetration in lab studies	Weak estrogen, moderate anti-androgen; associated with altered birthweight in human studies	Relatively high rates of skin allergy	N/A
Octinoxate (Octylmethoxycinnamate) Octinoxate, EMC, OMC, Ethylhexyl methoxycinnamate, Escalol 557, 2-Ethylhexyl-para-methoxycinnamate, Parsol MCX *Banned in Hawaii*	6 UVB only	Widespread *stabilizes* Avobenzone	Found in mothers' milk; less than 1% skin penetration in human and laboratory studies	Hormone-like activity; reproductive system, thyroid, and behavioral alterations in animal studies	Moderate rates of skin allergy	N/A

Chemical or Mineral	EWG Hazard Score	Use in U.S. Sunscreens and filter type	Skin Penetration	Hormone disruption	Skin Allergy	Other Concerns
Homosalate Homomethyl salicylate, HMS	4 UVB only	Widespread	Found in mothers' milk; skin penetration less than 1% studies	Disrupts estrogen, androgen, and progesterone	N/A	Toxic breakdown products
Octisalate Ethylhexyl-paramethoxycinnamate, Parsol MCX, octyl salicylate	4 UVB only	Widespread stabilizes avobenzone	Skin penetration in lab studies	N/A	Rarely reported skin allergy	N/A
Octocrylene Eusolex OCR, Parsol 340, 2-Cyano-3,3-diphenyl acrylic acid, 2-ethylhexylester	3 UVB only	Widespread	Found in mothers' milk; skin penetration in lab studies	N/A	Relatively high rates of skin allergy	N/A
Titanium Dioxide C177891 TO(2)	2 UVA/UVB	Widespread	No finding of skin penetration	No evidence hormone disruption	None	Inhalation concerns

Chemical or Mineral	EWG Hazard Score	Use in U.S. Sunscreens and filter type	Skin Penetration	Hormone disruption	Skin Allergy	Other Concerns
Zinc Oxide	2 UVA/UVB	Widespread; excellent protection	Less than 0.01% skin penetration in human volunteers	No evidence hormone disruption	None	Inhalation concerns
Avobenzone 1-(4-methoxyphenyl)-3-(4-tert-butyl phenyl) propane-1,3-dione, Butyl methoxy dibenzoylmethane, DBM, Parsol 1789, Eusolex 9020	2 UVA	Widespread; best protection of chemical filters	Limited skin penetration	No evidence hormone disruption	Breakdown product causes relatively high rates of skin allergy	Unstable in sunshine; must be mixed with stabilizers
Ecamsule Mexoryl SX, Terephthalylidene Dicamphor Sulfonic Acid	2 UVA	Uncommon; pending FDA approval; stable UVA protection	Less than 0.16% skin penetration in human volunteers	No evidence of hormone disruption	Skin allergy is rare	N/A

The best and least toxic chemical available today is Mexoryl, or ecamsule; however, it is not yet available in the United States as of this writing. Additional chemicals that are approved in Europe that are not approved by the FDA as of this writing may also have a low hazard score. One of these chemicals is Bisoctrizole. Presently, it is approved to use in UPF-rated clothing (Tinosorb), but not for sunscreen use.

Zinc oxide is the best and safest option. Also, you can now purchase sunscreens to match your skin tone. That said, for special occasions, using other low-hazard chemicals is an option for some.

Note that avobenzone and Mexoryl SX have a number 2 rating for the top-rated chemicals. However, they only protect against UVA rays, so if you use a product with either chemical, the product will have additional chemicals to block UVB rays.

Other Concerns Regarding Sunscreen Ingredients

This next section is about some of the other concerns regarding sunscreen products. It first covers a deeper exploration of estrogen-mimicking chemicals, which is then followed by safety concerns about the particle size of mineral ingredients.

The Problem with Endocrine Disrupting Chemicals

In the chart above, there is a column rating sunscreen chemicals for estrogenic activity. Estrogen-mimicking chemicals negatively impact the endocrine system, and they can alter normal hormonal functioning in our bodies and the bodies of animals. Many animal studies have shown that these chemicals can affect reproduction and development in males and females by altering reproductive and thyroid hormones. Animal studies report lower sperm counts and sperm abnormalities, altered menstrual cycling for female mice, and a

Danish study reported in 2016 that eight out of thirteen chemical sunscreen ingredients allowed in the United States affected calcium signaling of male sperm cells in laboratory tests, which the researchers suggest could reduce male fertility.

In 2018, Hawaii took the step to protect their coral reef. A 2015 study of coral reefs in Hawaii, the U.S. Virgin Islands, and Israel determined oxybenzone "leaches the coral of its nutrients and bleaches it white. It can also disrupt the development of fish and other wildlife." Even a small drop is enough to damage delicate corals.

Researchers have estimated that about 14,000 tons of sunscreen lotions end up in coral reefs around the world each year. Hawaii outlawed the chemicals oxybenzone and octinoxate, which are used in more than 3,500 of the world's most popular sunscreen products, including Hawaiian Tropic, Coppertone, and Banana Boat, which are now prohibited.

Mineral Particle-Size Safety: Nanoparticles and Micronized

Nanoparticles are super-finely ground zinc or titanium used in sunscreen to render it clear or invisible so that it is aesthetically more pleasing. Mineral sunscreens offer many advantages over chemical sunscreens, but some can have one drawback: appearance. Because they contain minerals (zinc oxide and/or titanium dioxide) that are meant to sit on top of the skin, these sunscreens can have a whitish appearance.

Some small studies have raised concerns regarding the potential toxicity of nanoparticles and suggest that they can cross the skin barrier into the bloodstream. More recent studies show that this is not likely. However, the EWG noted that the larger particle size of minerals does a better job of reflecting UV rays. My recommendation for the best overall protection is zinc oxide that states "micronized" or "non-nano." Some additional thoughts:

- Zinc oxide non-nano is the best and safest active ingredient.
- Look for products that offer micronized rather than nano-sized for the best UVB and, especially, UVA protection.
- Mineral products that use the word *clear* typically mean nanosized.
- Tinted mineral products are now available that more easily blend in with an individual's skin color.
- While micronized is overall best, using nano-sized has the benefit of a better appearance. For my sun-protection, I do use a nano-sized product for my face with a color to match my skin tone. For the rest of my body, I use micronized. Unfortunately, not all labels add this information.

The Best Solution: Mineral Sunscreen: Mineral sunscreen wins hands down in the competition to protect your skin from sunburn, especially given the many problems associated with chemical sunscreens (as discussed above). Zinc oxide offers full-spectrum protection without the additional use of multiple chemicals, which are potentially carcinogenic or hormone disrupting. Titanium runs a close second to zinc, but it is still not as effective as zinc.

It is better than most other active ingredients.

While no product is perfect, the next sections discuss some of the pros and cons of titanium dioxide and zinc oxide, as well as the issue of mineral coatings.

Titanium Dioxide Safety:

- Titanium has been utilized in foods, including gum, toothpaste, and almost anything that is white. Multiple studies have shown that it is safe to eat.

- Titanium dust that is inhaled may increase the risk of lung cancer. This is a finding of workers in manufacturing plants that were not wearing respirators to protect their lungs. As a lotion, there is no problem with inhaling particles.

Zinc Oxide Safety:

- According to Occupational Safety Health and Administration (OSHA), topical administration of zinc oxide on rabbits, mice, and guinea pigs failed to cause either skin irritation or signs of systemic toxicity.
- Factory workers exposed to zinc dust particles experienced temporary lung problems.

Nano-Particles and Mineral Coatings

According to EWG, it is unlikely that nanoparticles in sunscreen cause skin damage when energized by sunlight. Titanium dioxide, and to a lesser extent zinc oxide, are photocatalysts, meaning that when they are exposed to UV radiation, they can form free radicals that damage surrounding cells. Nanoparticle sizes of these minerals are more affected by UV rays than larger particles.

Sunscreen manufacturers commonly employ surface coatings that can dramatically reduce the potential for photoactivity, with data suggesting that they reduce UV reactivity by as much as 99 percent. In sunscreens, problems may arise if particles are not treated with inert coatings, if the coatings are not stable, or if manufacturers use forms of zinc oxide or titanium dioxide that are not optimized for stability and sun protection. However, tests of living skin from human volunteers and animal testing suggest that these hazards are not a concern for human safety because the free radicals that are generated by nanoparticles on skin are quenched by the skin's own antioxidant protections.

Allergens

Have you ever noticed that some chemical sunscreens are marketed as being "hypoallergenic"? That is because an itchy, blistering rash (known as "contact dermatitis") results when certain substances come in contact with the skin—and chemical sunscreens can contain some of those substances. Some manufacturers market their products as hypoallergenic because they should, theoretically, be less likely to cause an allergic reaction. But as with other issues regarding confusing labeling of sun protection products, the term *hypoallergenic* does not guarantee that you will not have a reaction to the product.

Some people have problems because of the active ingredients in a chemical sunscreen, but an allergic reaction may also be triggered by the fragrances, preservatives, or other ingredients in a product. In addition, the stress of being out in the sun, in very hot conditions, can exacerbate any rash. Further, anything that clogs the pores, such as products that contain waxes or petroleum ingredients, add to the potential for an allergic reaction.

Some people believe that the sun itself is the cause of a rash, rather than the sun-protection product being used, or the lotion put on his or her skin that day. I recall that a friend of mine spent much of her vacation in the shade, believing she was "allergic to the sun." When she stopped using her chemical sunscreen, the rash healed, and she was able to enjoy the rest of her vacation. In another instance, a friend developed a horrible rash and switched from her chemical sunscreen to a mineral product, and her rash resolved as well. Some individuals have excessively sensitive skin that can react to the heat of the sun's rays, resulting in skin rashes, but those instances are rarer.

Non-active ingredients to avoid

Listed below are some common non-active ingredients you should avoid. Not only are they unhealthy for humans but they also are often bad for the environment, too, including wildlife. Check the non-active ingredients list on sun protection products and avoid the ingredients listed below.

The Problem with Vitamin A

Vitamin A is an antioxidant, and it is still in many sunscreen products and body lotions, marketed as a substance that slows skin aging. However, studies have shown that vitamin A does result in oxidative damage when applied to the skin, including the lips.

Following is an excerpt from the EWG in 2018: "A study by U.S. government scientists suggests that retinyl palmitate, a form of vitamin A, may speed the development of skin tumors and lesions when applied to the skin in the presence of sunlight. Officials in Germany and Norway have cautioned that retinyl palmitate and other vitamin A ingredients in cosmetics could contribute to vitamin A toxicity due to excessive exposure."

- Parabens: In recent years, customer awareness of parabens has forced the cosmetic industry to find better preservatives. However, as of the writing of this book a reported 12 percent of cosmetic products still contain parabens, which has been shown to be "weakly" estrogenic. Don't be fooled by the term "weakly estrogenic." When you apply these substances frequently to your skin they accumulate. Eighteen different varieties of parabens exist, and you can easily spot them on most labels because they all contain the word "paraben" in their chemical nomenclature.

Toxicology studies links parabens to breast cancer in animal studies. Upon learning of the cancer-link possibility associated with parabens, I would warn against using underarm deodorant containing parabens, particularly as deodorant is applied daily from the teen years on throughout our lives. Allergic skin reaction to parabens is a known side effect. The risk of allergic reaction is especially common in sun-protection products because the heat of the sun exacerbates the reaction.

- Petroleum-Based Chemicals ("Estrogenic"): Petroleum-derived compounds (petrochemicals), including mineral oil, isopropyl alcohol, and more, are rated "weakly" estrogenic. Labels that include prefixes or suffixes such as: "methyl-," "propyl-," "-ene," or "-eth" are the clue that there is a petrochemical ingredient. Petroleum by-products are present in most lip products; "petrolatum" is mineral oil jelly.

- Mineral Oil: Mineral oil is petroleum based and is never recommended by health professionals who know anything about skin. Mineral oil is intended as a lubricant. But, instead of merely lubricating the skin, it blocks pores, thus interfering with the skin's ability to breathe and absorb moisture and nutrition. Furthermore, it disrupts the skin's natural immune barrier, making it more susceptible to skin conditions, including allergic reactions. Due to the drying effect and the disruption of natural body oil production, mineral oil contributes to the skin's premature aging. Ironically, mineral oil is an ingredient in many cosmetic products that we most closely associate with having a healing or therapeutic value, including baby oil, face and body lotion, sunscreen, and lipstick.

- Isopropyl Alcohol: Alcohol is a solvent and denaturant (a poisonous substance that changes another substance's natural qualities) that is found in hair-color rinses, body rubs, hand lotion, after-shave lotion, fragrances, and many other cosmetics and personal care products. Like mineral oil, iso-propyl alcohol is a petroleum-derived substance. It is a major ingredient in antifreeze and a solvent in shellac and diluted essential oils. Warning labels caution that ingestion or inhalation of the vapor may cause headaches, flushing, dizziness, mental depression, nausea, vomiting, narcosis, anesthesia, and coma.

Chemicals Can Contaminate Nature Too

Chemicals do not just disappear once they are used; eventually they end up in the environment where many have been found to negatively impact wildlife. It is sad and infuriating that a plethora of endocrine-disrupting chemicals have been released into the environment, and hundreds of new chemicals are added each year.

- Mercury: Even at low levels, mercury can damage brain function; so why, in these so-called enlightened times, are they still used in cosmetics? The preservative "thimerosal" contains some mercury.
- Fragrance: Fragrances fall into a colossal loophole in federal law that doesn't require companies to list on product labels any of the potentially hundreds of chemicals in a single product's fragrance mixture, says the EWG. Because fragrances can contain neurotoxins and are among the top five allergens ever, the EWG recommends we "vote with our pocketbooks" and steadfastly refuse to buy any artificially scented product.

Fragrances can come from more than 1,500 different chemicals, and many have been shown to exhibit hormonal activity, including the popular scent, musk.

- Herbs: Herbs are nature's medicines, and two of the most popular herbs are lavender and tea tree oil. Both have phytoestrogens that mimic the hormone estrogen. Soy is also a rich source. A few small studies linked breast growth in boys (gynecomastia) and early breast growth in girls as young as four or five who used products with these two herbs. Some studies contradicted these findings. Bottom line, I do not recommend long-term daily use of either herb on the skin for children, or adults, especially those that exhibit estrogenic activity. Short-term use is fine.

How to Use Sun Protection Products Effectively

Smart consumers not only have to read labels, they must also seek out reputable companies. In general, if you do not recognize an ingredient, choose a different product. When shopping for skin products, your best bet is health food stores, if you are savvy. But even in health food stores you must be vigilant, as you will find many products that contain substances on the do-not-buy list mentioned above. Definitely familiarize yourself with the resource Environmental Working Group (EWG) online to look up current findings regarding ingredients in the products you purchase. Also, EWG is giving its seal of approval to products that meet the organization's standards for healthy ingredients.

Guide for effective sunscreen use: Not enough people are using sun protection products or smart strategies to avoid too much sun exposure. Here's what you can do to make sure your sunscreen works right for you:

- Make sure when you apply sunscreen that you apply what the label recommends.
- Read the active and inactive ingredient lists and make sure, if you are using the best-rated mineral (zinc oxide) that the percentage is at least 20 percent for an SPF 30 protection. Zinc is the best for both UVA and UVB protection.
- Preferably buy mineral products that are labeled non-nano or micronized size.
- Use a generous amount of sunscreen product on exposed skin—at least one ounce per application, or more depending on body size. Most sunscreens today are lotions. When you put it on it should be thick; let it soak in and then spread the rest evenly. To help you determine what one ounce is, a shot glass is 1.5 ounces.
- Do not forget to apply sunscreen to sensitive areas, particularly the top of the ears, back of the neck, the nose, and the top of shoulders and feet.
- Apply sunscreen approximately twenty to thirty minutes before going out into the sun.
- Re-apply sunscreen frequently in intense sun situations and when sweating or swimming.
- Look for "reef safe" on the label.
- Water-resistant labeling must pass independent tests to prove they retain their stated SPF while swimming or sweating. Labels must now state 40 minutes or 80 minutes of water-resistance. The term *waterproof* is no longer allowed by the FDA.
- Do not rub sun protection products into your skin because, especially with minerals, the product should essentially sit on top of the surface of your skin in order to reflect and block UV rays.

- When applying lotion, smooth it on your skin. Wait fifteen to thirty seconds and gently smooth out the remaining lotion. Many mineral products become less visible after fifteen to twenty minutes following application, as it blends into the skin.
- Make sure you are putting into practice safe and mindful sun-protection strategies for you and your family on a daily basis.
- Don't be misled by advertising. Read product labels carefully!
- Expiration date—recycle if the product is more than two years old or if you can see that it is separating when you put it on your skin. Products that are kept in hot climates will not last as long. If the sunscreen appears to separate dispose of it.

Sports and Sun Protection

The best strategy for protecting you and your family from too much sun while participating in sports is to use UPF-rated clothing to cover your skin whenever possible and put chemical-free sunscreen on areas that are not covered. Maintaining protection from the sun while swimming can be challenging for two reasons: sunscreens come off in water and thus require frequent reapplication. One of the best protections for swimmers is to avoid swimming between 10 a.m. and 3 p.m., especially in tropical regions. That advice also holds for people going on vacation in hot climates who want to avoid the painful sunburns that could ruin a trip.

Vote with Your Wallet

As you have learned in this chapter, commercial personal care products contain chemicals that have a real health impact, because what we put on our skin has the very real possibility of ending up in our bloodstream. As the body's largest organ, skin is very permeable. On a personal level, we can limit our own exposure to these harmful chemicals by educating ourselves, and by buying only products we are assured are chemical free. The larger issue is political; in the voting booth, I personally endorse and support leaders on every governmental level who have shown a commitment to keeping our environment clean and safe, and a willingness to advocate for a better-regulated cosmetic industry. At the drug store and supermarket, I cast a "vote" with my wallet by not purchasing chemical-laden products, and by supporting the manufacturers of pure, safe products.

In the final chapter, the focus is on the health benefits of sunlight itself, beyond the UV rays. The seasons of the year and the length of daylight guide our internal clock or circadian rhythm, and this is critical for our overall health.

Key Points from Chapter 12 — Safe Sunscreens and Chemicals to Avoid

- Proper sunscreen use can reduce future skin cancers.

- Don't be fooled by high SPF.

- Avoid products with vitamin A—it may speed the development of some skin cancers.

- Zinc oxide is the best active ingredient for both UVA and UVB protection

- Many chemicals that are used in sunscreens exhibit hormonal activity

- Some chemicals have been banned in areas where coral reefs grow

- You must apply the recommended amount of sunscreen

- SPF 30 is 97% protection from UVB rays

Chapter 13:

Sunlight, Darkness, and Circadian Rhythm

> Circadian rhythm (popular name is bio-rhythm): The "internal body clock" that regulates the twenty-four-hour cycle of biological processes in animals and plants. *Circa* (Latin), meaning "around" and *dies* meaning "day"—literally, around a day.

Let there be light! Many of us who work indoors are not getting enough natural sunlight to support our innate biological rhythm. For millions of years, plants and animals have lived with sunlight and have adapted to it. Most plants exposed only to incandescent or florescent light will not thrive. Is it possible that humans, too, are "wilting" in the indoor world we've adapted to? We are meant to take natural sunlight in through our eyes, and that light affects multiple body functions.

The seasons of the year and the length of daylight guide our internal clock, which is also known as circadian rhythm. Mammals are hardwired to respond to shorter or longer daylight hours. Animals that hibernate, such as bears, know exactly when to begin to look for their winter sleeping place. During hibernation, they suspend the search for food, they stop eating, their body temperature drops, and their metabolism slows, thus minimizing the animal's energy output and allowing it to live until spring on the fat stored from summer's and fall's high consumption. Spring's lengthening daylight signals the animal that it is time to emerge—hungry, thinner, ready to hunt, and ready to perpetuate the new year's cycle once more.

Without artificial light sources, our ancestors went to sleep soon after sunset and rose near sunrise. But with the advent of electric light came the option to stay awake much later than nature intended. In essence, we have created an "endless summer" in terms of the ratio of hours awake to hours asleep. But the problem is that we human mammals are still programmed to sleep longer hours, conserve energy, and eat less during winter months. We are not living in harmony with our nature in today's world of active engagement after dark and far past what would be our natural "bedtime." Regardless of what our mammal nature craves, most people do not have the means or the desire to replicate the schedule of our cave-dwelling ancestors. So, the problem for us, with our hardwired circadian rhythm, is how to make peace with and stay healthy in the "city that never sleeps" world in which we now live.

All Light Is Not Created Equal

Indoor lighting does not duplicate sunlight—ever! Full-spectrum, natural sunlight includes the visible light that we can see, as well as non-visible light. There are several crucial differences between indoor lighting and natural lighting. The luminosity of indoor light is different (brightness) from sunlight. Fluorescent bulbs that emit only the blue spectrum are now strongly promoted as environmentally, and economically, the right choice for light bulbs with which to light our homes. But, unfortunately, fluorescent bulbs emit an unnatural light and have been linked to skin cancer and other illnesses. The newer full-spectrum light bulbs are a huge improvement over older fluorescent bulbs, but still, they are not the same as natural light. Halogen bulbs also emit UV rays and should be covered. Bulbs made today come with a thick glass cover. There are better and worse choices for us to make in our homes and any other artificially lighted places in which we can exercise control, or at least influence.

Sunlight and Our Health

Mal-illumination is a term coined by the late light-science pioneer, John Ott. He referred to mal-illumination as a "silent epidemic" and likened it to malnutrition. The condition of mal-illumination is now widely accepted as a health risk for our artificially lit world. We require the full spectrum of sunlight energy for the development and maintenance of a healthy body. John Ott also developed full-spectrum light technology, which you will read about later in this chapter.

When we are able to live in concert with the natural cycles of sunlight and darkness, our bodies are "in sync." Although we can't and wouldn't want to bring back a schedule of ending our activities and readying ourselves for sleep at dusk, it is important for our health to develop good habits to support our circadian rhythm. One way to do this is to venture outdoors every day. While this may not be practical during extreme weather conditions, it is how our ancestors lived out of necessity. When we do make the effort to balance our natural biorhythms, by exposing ourselves to daylight, every day, and sleeping in the dark, we will be rewarded with a deeper restorative sleep cycle, and a more alert wakefulness during daylight hours. Other benefits of maintaining a healthy circadian rhythm are:

- Cancer protection
- Normal sleep cycles
- Healthy immune system
- Regulation of body weight
- Reproduction/fertility
- Mood and mental balance
- Heart health including blood pressure

- Energy regulation
- Digestive health

Sunlight and Melatonin Production

Melatonin regulates sleep. It is a hormone that is produced and secreted by the pineal gland (located in the center of the brain) in response to light and darkness. Melatonin production is stimulated by darkness and inhibited by light. Early morning light acts as a resetting mechanism by switching off melatonin, signaling daytime. Synthesis and secretion of melatonin is dramatically affected by light exposure to the eyes. The typical serum concentrations of melatonin are low during the daylight hours and increase to a peak during the dark. So, we can think of melatonin as a positive dark force.

Melatonin triggers the deep sleep known as the delta rhythm and with that regulates the body's circadian rhythm. As melatonin is also a powerful antioxidant, it plays a significant role in modulating immune function by acting against the most damaging free radical, the OH molecule (hydroxide), which causes oxidative damage. An example of oxidative damage is seen in an apple when it is cut open and exposed to ambient air; without the protection of the apple skin, the fruit surface soon turns brown. Unabated free-radical damage in our body hastens aging and causes or accelerates disease processes. So, in addition to eating vegetables and fruits to promote the production of antioxidants that support healthy aging, we can add melatonin into our arsenal of free-radical fighters.

Because we have extended "daylight" with artificial light after sunset, our pineal glands perceive a longer, extended "day time." This unnatural lengthening of day can result in undesirable health consequences—most notably sleep disturbances including insomnia because with less "night time" there is less opportunity for the body to produce the melatonin it needs for optimal sleep inducement.

Production of melatonin is naturally higher earlier in life, peaking in puberty and very gradually declining as we age. Some people have abnormally low levels of melatonin, which in part may be due to our modern, abnormal light exposure. Ongoing, unremitting high levels of stress can also lead to an abnormally low melatonin level.

As we have just learned, sunlight and artificial light impact our natural production of melatonin. Our lifestyle and diet also play a role in melatonin production. For example, tryptophan is an amino acid that we get from our diet that can be converted into serotonin and melatonin. Tryptophan and the other molecules it produces influences many functions in the body, including sleep, mood, and behavior.

Melatonin Supplementation

Supplementation of melatonin is primarily used for three health issues; sleep disturbances, jet lag, and less frequently, cancer treatment. There is concern that supplementation of melatonin could disrupt the body's ability to produce melatonin naturally, which in turn might negatively affect the pineal gland. Some researchers do caution against regular use of melatonin. On the other hand, alternative cancer clinics often prescribe 6 mg or more of melatonin to fight cancer. As usual, in the world of health care, there are conflicting opinions.

When evaluating opposing treatment modalities, it is a good idea to consider and weigh all views, then, when possible, choose the treatment that is in accord with what is most natural. In the case of melatonin, it is best to optimize natural melatonin production by increasing exposure to natural daylight and decreasing nighttime exposure of artificial light. However, if you want to try supplementation .5 mg, under the tongue (sublingual), is a reasonable place to start to see if it is helpful. Some people report disturbed sleep on doses of 3 mg, including nightmares.

Your melatonin levels can be tested with a blood test, urine test, or saliva test. If you are concerned that you may actually be melatonin deficient, ask your doctor about testing. Melatonin is produced by the pineal gland and sends a signal to regulate the sleep-wake cycle in the sleep center of the brain. Interestingly, melatonin is also produced in the retina, the skin, and the GI tract, but this is not the melatonin that affects your biological sleep clock.

Increasing Natural Sunlight for Our Health and Melatonin Production

It is important for our health to develop habits that facilitate restoring our natural circadian rhythm as much as possible. Here are some simple solutions to incorporate more natural sunlight during daytime hours, as well as some strategies for dealing with indoor lighting to help your brain prepare for sleep. These suggestions will help you establish a more natural circadian rhythm, which in turn will facilitate increased melatonin production.

- Allow your eyes to take in sunlight, especially before 10:00 a.m. (the earlier the better), for a minimum of ten minutes, and longer if possible. Direct sunlight in the eyes is not recommended, so wear a hat or hang out in the shade for ambient light.
- Whenever possible, step outside to enjoy reading, writing, or participating in any activity that allows you to be outside. How much time is necessary to reap the benefits? As much as possible, but at least an hour throughout the day would be best. Sitting in the shade on sunny days counts too.
- Sit by open windows when possible. Glass filters out some of the natural light.
- If you work in a large office building, do your best to take breaks outside.

- Don't wear sunglasses every time you are outside. When necessary, protect your eyes and allow your eyes to take in ambient light, especially during morning hours. Even that walk to the car is a moment when you can get natural light.
- Use soft indoor lighting after sunset. Energy-conscious people have switched their softer incandescent bulbs for florescent bulbs. Use fluorescent bulbs for household areas that you do not frequent during nighttime, including closets and all outdoor lighting.
- Turn off devices early that produce unnatural light, such as cell phones, computers, and televisions.
- Sleep in a darkened room.
- Go to sleep as soon after sunset as possible—I acknowledge that given our modern lifestyle this is nearly impossible for most of us.
- Turn off electronic devices early in the evening. This includes mobile phones, computers and televisions.
- Prudent avoidance of light at night will help ensure normal levels of melatonin, whether we work night shifts or not. Dim those lights!

Now that we have learned how to improve getting enough safe sunlight to assist our circadian rhythm, the next section deals with how significant lack of sunlight may result in health conditions.

Should you Expose your Eyes Directly to Sunlight?

There are many recommendations that you may read in articles or online. Some suggest 20-30 minutes, or more, of morning sunshine, directly into the eyes or with eyes closed. UVA rays are strong all day. UVB rays are not present or they are weak in early morning hours. UVA can damage your central vision. It can damage the macula, a part of the retina at the back of your eyes. Since UVA rays penetrate deeply, closing the eyes will not protect the inner eyes.

UVB rays mostly damage the cornea and lens. Therefore, until I see a definitive study regarding the safety of direct sunlight into the eyes my recommendation is non-direct bright ambient light for 20-30 minutes, before 10:00 am or earlier. Wearing a hat or standing under an umbrella when the light is bright is safe and recommended in early morning hours.

Conditions That Are Associated with Lack of Sunlight

Significant research points to health problems that can result when our circadian rhythm is disturbed. It is well known that those who regularly work night shift hours are subject to many conditions that have been associated with an upset in their normal rhythm. Ambient sunlight taken in through our eyes has many health benefits and directly impacts our natural circadian rhythm. Even birds, especially hawks, take in sunlight through their eyes, which improves their vision. Following are some of the common conditions that are associated with lack of sunlight exposure or circadian rhythm disruption.

Insomnia

Insomnia is a widespread and serious condition. Sleeping is restorative and allows our bodies the needed rejuvenation. Sleep deprivation causes decreased brain function. When tested, people who are deprived of sleep cannot perform as well as those who are rested, resulting in impaired judgment, problem solving, and physical coordination. In fact, tiredness can be as dangerous as drunkenness on our roadways. Ongoing lack of sleep is stressful and can lead to a weakened immune system.

Too often the "solution" to complaints of insomnia have been the prescription of sleep-inducing drugs, which are not only habit forming but produce a quality of sleep that does not replicate natural or restorative sleep. Instead, the drugs often leave the sleeper groggy and dream-deprived. For those who are plagued with insomnia, it is particularly important to consider the role of sunlight and melatonin production in order to improve sleeping patterns.

Most of us go through periods of lack of sleep. One night is easy to recover from. However, studies show that multiple nights of sleeplessness is as dangerous as alcohol when it comes to driving an automobile. Hormone imbalance, health conditions, and lifestyle issues play a huge role in sleep problems for many people. If you suffer from ongoing sleep deprivation you may need to see a sleep specialist. It is also important to work with a doctor that practices holistic medicine that includes nutrition and hormone balancing.

When natural treatments do not work, medications may be needed. For instance, depression and insomnia often go together, and a medication may be necessary to break the pattern. Or, there could be an underlying health problem such as hypothyroidism. This is why it is important to have a health evaluation from a doctor familiar with providing a complete health assessment.

Body Weight and Sunlight

We learned in Chapter 5 that vitamin D deficiency has been linked to weight gain and obesity. An additional reason for the prevalence of obesity may be explained by a theory posited by John Ott, investigator of groundbreaking research on the effects of full-spectrum light on plants, animals, and humans. Ott's research showed that mammals are programmed by the length of day and seasons of the year: they eat less and sleep longer during darker, winter months. Though this was long known about hibernating animals, Ott's work carries this reasoning to humans, suggesting that the partial answer to obesity may be found in our electrically lit world. Artificial light has effectively extended the length of our days to mimic the long summer days that our forbearers lived, which was necessary to build up their fat stores that they would need during the short winter period. Humans have lengthened their winter days with artificial light. As a result, our bodies behave as though these long days are like summer. So, we eat as if it's summer year-round!

John Ott's findings were originally met with polite indifference from the scientific community, but he began to attract attention from a wider public with his theory of mal-illumination. Much of Ott's work has been validated by subsequent research, and his contribution to our Much of Ott's work has been validated by subsequent research, and his contribution to our understanding of how light interacts with our physiology is acknowledged by experts and professionals across the spectrum.

Depression

Sunlight stimulates serotonin production, the hormone that gives us that wonderful sense of well-being. As a neurotransmitter, serotonin is a major component of healthy brain chemistry and a precursor for melatonin synthesis. Some studies have shown that serotonin production is also stimulated by skin exposure to sunlight. So, now we have a scientific explanation for why sunbathing makes us feel so-o-o-o good! Sunlight is crucial for mental health, and it is overlooked by most conventional medical doctors as a consideration when treating depression.

Most medications prescribed for depression today target serotonin in some way. The most commonly prescribed medications that treat depression are in a category of drugs called serotonin uptake inhibitors, or SSRIs. Their action is implied in the name—they inhibit the uptake in the tissues of serotonin, and therefore increase the blood level of serotonin. SSRI medications have been undeniably helpful for many people suffering debilitating depression. While SSRIs are a wise choice for serious depression, they tend to be overprescribed, as so many medications are. Conventional medicine often overlooks the importance of natural medicine. Over the years I have witnessed many patients resolve depression by focusing on exercise and nutrition that includes vitamin D and sunlight treatment programs. Medications have their place; however, a balanced diet, exercise, and sunlight should always be the cornerstone for physical and mental health.

Seasonal Affective Disorder (SAD)

Seasonal affective disorder, or SAD, is a well-accepted syndrome that occurs in fall and winter in northern countries due to light deficiency in winter months. It has been estimated that up to 10 percent of people living in Alaska and New Hampshire suffer from SAD. The most common age of onset is in the thirties. Symptoms include:

- depression in winter months
- low energy levels during the day
- diminished general sense of well-being
- difficulty sleeping
- fatigue
- social withdrawal
- excessive sleeping
- overeating
- carbohydrate craving
- weight gain

The following excerpt from a study indicates that light itself can be a sole source for serotonin release by the brain.

"The rate of production of serotonin by the brain was directly related to the prevailing duration of bright sunlight and rose rapidly with increased luminosity. Our findings are further evidence for the notion that changes in release of serotonin by the brain underlie mood seasonality and seasonal affective disorder."

As mentioned in Chapter 5, vitamin D deficiency has been linked to depression. Depression and mood disorders are complex and require clinicians to consider each case on its own merits; however, sunlight exposure to increase vitamin D stores as well as regularly allowing our eyes to take in the full-spectrum natural ambient light are treatments to consider.

Light Therapy for the Treatment of SAD: Small, portable light devices have been developed for the treatment of SAD. These devices are also recommended for treatment of other conditions such as sleep disorders, jet lag, dementia, types of depression that don't occur seasonally, and adjusting to a nighttime work schedule.

The lightbox contains a specific type of fluorescent bulbs or tubes. The bulbs are covered with a plastic screen that helps block out potentially harmful ultraviolet (UVA) rays that can cause cataracts and skin problems. The treatment consists of the patient sitting for a specified period of time each day near the box so that the box's light strikes the patient's skin. As with every treatment program, there are questions regarding safety. Apparently, some people have damaged their eyes by either using the box incorrectly or by using a poorly constructed unit.

The quality and type of bulb is of utmost importance if light treatment is to be both safe and effective. Light boxes are fairly expensive, but the bulbs in a lightbox emit an intensity of light that isn't found in household lighting. Simply sitting in front of your living room lamp cannot relieve the symptoms of SAD. Is it possible to build your own box? It is! But, before you do, I suggest you visit the Mayo Clinic website (www.mayoclinic.org) because not all lightboxes are created equal. And, there are contraindications for some people who have certain mental disorders. Also, side effects, especially when not administered correctly, include eyestrain, headaches, and nausea.

Some studies have reported increased levels of serotonin, dopamine, and possibly melatonin with consistent use of a lightbox, and a general sense of well-being, enhanced by exposure to the box's bright light.

Fertility and Light

The importance of light is usually overlooked by doctors when they are exploring the inability to conceive. Perhaps sunlight, together with vitamin D, is the answer some couples are looking for. This may seem too simple a solution in today's world of in vitro fertilization, but many animal studies indicate the importance of vitamin D, melatonin, and sunlight itself in reproduction.

A study using hamsters demonstrated that a hamster that does not have a pineal gland does not prepare for the breeding season. In addition, the research showed that a pineal gland unable to receive photo/light information would not function. These studies are far from conclusive proof of a direct causal relationship between insufficient light and infertility, but the implication is certainly suggestive.

PMS and Light

A small study of twenty women who suffered from PMS used a lightbox for a four-month period. Their serotonin production increased, and their PMS symptoms were dramatically reduced. This study result is not entirely surprising as we know that male and female hormone levels are tied to sunlight exposure and vitamin D production.

Cancer and the Effects of Imbalanced Light and Darkness

One study demonstrated that melatonin has the ability to slow tumor growth up to 70 percent in mice infected with human breast cancer cells. When the mice were subjected to constant light, cancer growth rocketed. (Remember, our bodies produce melatonin during dark hours.) Yet, another study found that mice with breast cancer cells could slow the tumor growth with melatonin supplementation.

Other studies have explored the connection between our relationship to light, dark, and cancer. An ongoing study of eighty-thousand female nurses conducted at Brigham Young University and the Women's Hospital in Boston reported that nurses who worked night shifts at least three times a month, for a period of fifteen years or more, were 35 percent more likely to develop colorectal cancer than those who worked mostly day shifts. Breast cancer has also been linked to nightshift workers, likely due to low levels of melatonin. Nightshift workers have higher risks for many illnesses, including cancers, heart disease, and mental disorders. In addition to having lower levels of melatonin, nightshift workers widely use caffeine and nicotine in an effort to stay awake, which increases stress levels, another known risk factor for cancer. Vitamin D deficiency is more common in nightshift workers than those that work day shifts.

These findings suggest that the combined stressors mentioned above sets up a perfect environment for cancers to develop and grow. Simply put, the immune system becomes overtaxed, to the breaking point. While we often can't control which shift we work, we can use what we know about the importance of getting the right balance between more natural light and dark (for sleeping) to mitigate against those stressors we can control. Of course, cutting back on the caffeine and quitting smoking is, as always, going to be part of every cancer-reduction effort for all of us.

Full-Spectrum Home and Office Lighting

I highly recommend the use of full-spectrum lighting in the home, and at work, too, if that is possible to arrange. Full-spectrum halogen and fluorescent bulbs are available where light bulbs are sold. They are more expensive to buy, but they last longer than incandescent bulbs. It is definitely worth the investment. If you work under a fluorescent bulb, try to have it removed and replaced with a freestanding lamp or full-spectrum bulbs. If your employer will not foot the bill, consider changing it yourself. Your health will benefit and maybe your mood at work will too!

Sunglasses Impair Circadian Rhythm

Wearing sunglasses all the time can throw off our circadian rhythm. If you want to keep the sun out of your eyes, and enjoy some ambient light, wear a hat that also protects your face from direct UV exposure. The pupil of the eye reacts to bright light by contracting and becoming smaller, thereby letting in less light, which protects the inner eye from increased damage. The lighter the eye color, the more the eye is subject to damage with prolonged, ongoing sun exposure. Sunglasses allow the pupil to relax and open wide to receive more light, so it is very important that you choose sunglasses that have full-spectrum protection from UVB and UVA. Early sunglasses did not filter UVA rays effectively and many of us were getting more eye damage from the unfiltered UVA rays.

Today, sunglasses are *supposed* to provide full-spectrum protection and should have a label with protection description. However, there are reports that some inexpensive sunglasses are not providing 100 percent UVB and UVA protection. At my optometrist's office they can check to see if my sunglasses provide what they advertise. You might want to have yours checked too.

Sunglasses are recommended under circumstances such as these:

- The sun is shining directly in your eyes.
- Anytime you find yourself squinting
- Glare is present; snow, water, and sand all increase UV intensity.
- You are in the mountains—high altitudes increase the intensity of UV radiation.
- You are driving in the city and there is high glare.

Another easy strategy for protecting the eyes is sun-shading hats, which you should always have available for when you need them. Carry hats in the car for all members of your family. The best color for sunglasses is gray, as it does not distort light as much as other colors.

Safe Sunlight for Healthy Eyes and More

The need to protect our eyes from too much harsh, intense sunlight is well-known and indisputable. There is clear evidence that people who live or work in consistent, extreme sun situations risk eye damage that may result in cataracts. Two examples that are often cited to support eye protection are fisherman and desert dwellers. Studies have found that in both situations, cataracts and even blindness are common later in life unless they can have cataract surgery.

However, there is no evidence that cautious, non-extreme sunlight exposure is harmful. The goal is to develop a mindful relationship with the sun. Obtaining the benefits of exposing our eyes to a reasonable amount of natural daylight plays an important role in our health. A mindful relationship with sunlight is to think of it as food for your eyes and circadian rhythm, making sure that several times a day you are outside in shaded light to benefit from the nourishment of ambient light. From what we have covered, we can appreciate how essential light is for our natural biorhythms, and it is clear that exposing the eyes to indirect natural sunlight is extremely important for our good health. Many books have been devoted to imparting this key message. Yet, this information is lost among the many messages about the dangers associated with sun exposure. As with everything I've covered in this chapter, the central issue to circadian rhythms and their impact on our bodily systems is balance—the balance between light exposure and darkness; the balance between the demands of living in a modern artificially lit world and respecting our primal need for rest and retreat; the balance between availing ourselves of the answers that technology offers and listening to, and relying on, timeless natural wisdom.

Key Points from Chapter 13 — Sunlight, Darkness, and Circadian Rhythm

- Live in concert with the natural cycles of sunlight and darkness, our bodies are "in sync"

- Allow your eyes to take in sunlight, especially before 10:00 a.m.

- Wear a hat or hang out in the shade for bright ambient light

- Sit by open windows when possible

- Use soft indoor lighting after sunset

- Turn off electronic devices early in the evening

- Sleep in a darkened room

- Melatonin is a powerful antioxidant

Conclusion

I wrote this book to help readers sort out the plethora of information regarding the sun; however, I also wanted to give all of my readers the information they need to safely interact with the sun. By the time I finished this book, I had had more than 20 diagnosed and treated skin cancers. And because of what I know, I caught them early, well before my dermatologist detected them. I was lucky, and they were easily treated. In short, I take very seriously the information that I share with readers because skin cancer can be avoided.

This book has shown you how to safely obtain vitamin D from the sun, as well as how to achieve optimal supplementation when needed. It has given you an overview of the factors that contribute to your particular risk of developing skin cancer, based on your skin type and family history. It also has provided strong recommendations regarding mineral and chemical sunscreens along with non-active ingredients to avoid, minimizing oxidative damage to the skin.

Our overall health depends on how we engage with the sun. In fact, if you learn only one thing from reading this book, I hope it is this: No one-size-fits-all approach exists when engaging with the sun. Each of us is unique, and because of this, we need to know our personal risks and benefits when exposing or not exposing our skin to the sun's rays.

The current medical approach for dealing with sun exposure can be one-dimensional; primarily, the medical community advises us to avoid the sun. In contrast, I've encouraged you to take the true complexity of our amazing sun into account, using an approach that is a mindful and conscious relationship. I've also asked you to maintain a healthy skepticism when it comes to testimonials and advertising of products for sun protection—and even skin cancer treatments—on the Internet. As you've learned, most skin cancers can be treated successfully with excellent results when they are caught early.

Skin health can be positively impacted at any time in life, if we choose to maintain a healthful lifestyle that includes exercise to increase muscle strength and balance. And remember, there will always be new information, because skin health research is ongoing.

Finally, as part of my attempt to give you an alternative and more integrative perspective on engaging with the sun, I've also emphasized the fact that, even if you have been diagnosed with skin cancer or you are in a high-risk skin cancer group, there is much you can do to reduce your risk for developing further skin damage, while developing a healthy relationship with the sun.

Despite conventional medicine's focus on avoiding sunburns and excessive sun exposure—a point with which I agree—the real name of the game is to view the skin from a broader perspective, purchasing healthy skin products, maintaining a healthful whole foods diet, and choosing a lifestyle that includes good nutrition and exercise to promote skin health.

Appendix

Skin Cancer Types

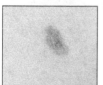

Actinic Keratosis—*Precancerous Growth*
Scaly crusty growths that form in areas most exposed to the sun: face, scalp, lips and back of hands.

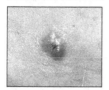

Atypical Moles—*Begnine Growths that Look Similar to Melanoma*
People who have atypical moles have an increased risk of developing Melanoma.

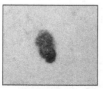

Merkel Cell Carncinoma—*Rare Aggressive Form of Skin Cancer*
This form of skin cancer has a high risk of recurring or spreading.

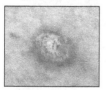

Melanoma—*The Deadliest Form of Skin Cancer*
Caiused mainly by UV exposure, or those who are genetically predisposed to the disease.

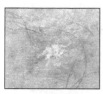

Squamous Cell Carcinoma—*Second Most Common Type of Skin Cancer*
Can appear on any part of the body, but typically forms in area exposed to the sun. Can be deadly if untreated.

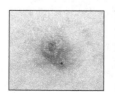

Basal Cell Carcinoma—*Most Common Type of Skin Cancer*
These growths form in the outermost layer of skin. This type of skin ca ncer generally never spreads to other parts.

MELANOMA

	Basal Cell Carcinoma (BCC)	Squamous Cell Carcinoma (SCC)	Melanoma
Appearance	• Flesh-colored pearl-like bump • Pinkish patch of skin	• Firm red bump • Scaly patch • Sore that does not fully heal	A mole that is asymmetrical, has an irregular border, multi-colored, 6mm or greater in diameter, changing (ABCDEs of Melanoma)
Where it appears	Typically on the head, neck & arms, but may appear anywhere.	Most common on the ears, face, neck, arms, chest and back.	Anywhere on the body, including nails or genital area.
Dangers	Can damage other tissue, including nerves & bones	Can damage other tissues including bone. May spread to lymph nodes or other parts of the body	Can metastasize and be fatal if not caught early.
Treatment	Excision or Mohs Surgery	Excision or Mohs Surgery	Excision or Mohs Surgery if caught *in situ* (Stage 0). More intensive treatment including chemo if in later stages.

www.beverlyskin.com

Bibliography

Alleviation of migraines with therapeutic vitamin D and calcium. Thys-Jacobs S. Headache. 1994 Nov-Dec;34(10):590-2. PubMed [citation] PMID: 7843955

Vitamin D and calcium in menstrual migraine. Thys-Jacobs S. Headache. 1994 Oct;34(9):544-6. PubMed [citation]PMID: 8002332

Vitamin D deficiency and otosclerosis. Brookes GB. Otolaryngol Head Neck Surg. 1985 Jun;93(3):313-21. PubMed [citation]PMID: 3927224

1,25-Dihydroxyvitamin D is not responsible for toxicity caused by vitamin D or 25-hydroxyvitamin D. Deluca HF, Prahl JM, Plum LA. Arch Biochem Biophys. 2011 Jan 15;505(2):226-30. doi: 10.1016/j.abb.2010.10.012. Epub 2010 Oct 18. PubMed [citation] PMID: 20965147

1Serum 25-hydroxyvitamin D concentrations in obese and non-obese women with polycystic ovary syndrome. Yildizhan R, Kurdoglu M, Adali E, Kolusari A, Yildizhan B, Sahin HG, Kamaci M. Arch Gynecol Obstet. 2009 Oct;280(4):559-63. doi: 10.1007/s00404-009-0958-7. Epub 2009 Feb 13. PubMed [citation]PMID: 19214546

Association of hypovitaminosis D with metabolic disturbances in polycystic ovary syndrome. Wehr E, Pilz S, Schweighofer N, Giuliani A, Kopera D, Pieber TR, Obermayer-Pietsch B. Eur J Endocrinol. 2009 Oct;161(4):575-82. doi: 10.1530/EJE-09-0432. Epub 2009 Jul 23. PubMed [citation]PMID: 19628650

Basal cell carcinoma: histological classification and body-site distribution. Raasch BA, Buettner PG, Garbe C. Br J Dermatol. 2006 Aug;155(2):401-7. PubMed [citation]PMID: 16882181

Calcium and vitamin D intake and risk of incident premenstrual syndrome. Bertone-Johnson ER, Hankinson SE, Bendich A, Johnson SR, Willett WC, Manson JE. Arch Intern Med. 2005 Jun 13;165(11):1246-52. PubMed [citation]PMID: 15956003

Calcium, vitamin D and cancer. Peterlik M, Grant WB, Cross HS. Anticancer Res. 2009 Sep;29(9):3687-98. Review. PubMed [citation] PMID: 19667166

Cancer prevention by tea: Evidence from laboratory studies. Yang CS, Wang H, Li GX, Yang Z, Guan F, Jin H. Pharmacol Res. 2011 Aug;64(2):113-22. doi: 10.1016/j.phrs.2011.03.001. Epub 2011 Mar 21. Review. PubMed [citation]PMID: 21397027

Changes in vitamin D metabolites during teriparatide treatment. Cosman F, Dawson-Hughes B, Wan X, Krege JH. Bone. 2012 Jun;50(6):1368-71. doi: 10.1016/j.bone.2012.02.635. Epub 2012 Mar 9. PubMed [citation]PMID: 22426307

Dietary vitamin D intake, 25-hydroxyvitamin D3 levels and premenstrual syndrome in a college-aged population. Bertone-Johnson ER, Chocano-Bedoya PO, Zagarins SE, Micka AE, Ronnenberg AG. J Steroid Biochem Mol Biol. 2010 Jul;121(1-2):434-7. doi: 10.1016/j.jsbmb.2010.03.076. Epub 2010 Apr 14. PubMed [citation] PMID: 20398756

Does D matter? The role of vitamin D in hair disorders and hair follicle cycling. Amor KT, Rashid RM, Mirmirani P. Dermatol Online J. 2010 Feb 15;16(2):3. Review. PubMed [citation]PMID: 20178699

Effect of treatment with dydrogesterone or calcium plus vitamin D on the severity of premenstrual syndrome. Khajehei M, Abdali K, Parsanezhad ME, Tabatabaee HR. Int J Gynaecol Obstet. 2009 May;105(2):158-61. doi: 10.1016/j.ijgo.2009.01.016. Epub 2009 Feb 20. PubMed [citation]PMID: 19232611

Epidemiology of vitamin D and colorectal cancer: casual or causal link? Giovannucci E. J Steroid Biochem Mol Biol. 2010 Jul;121(1-2):349-54. doi: 10.1016/j.jsbmb.2010.03.085. Epub 2010 Apr 14. Review. PubMed [citation]PMID: 20398758

From the bench to emerging new clinical concepts: Our present understanding of the importance of the vitamin D endocrine system (VDES) for skin cancer. Trémezaygues L, Reichrath J. Dermatoendocrinol. 2011 Jan;3(1):11-7. doi: 10.4161/derm.3.1.14875. PubMed [citation] PMID: 21519403 PMCID: PMC3051847

Functions of vitamin D in bone. Goltzman D. Histochem Cell Biol. 2018 Apr;149(4):305-312. doi: 10.1007/s00418-018-1648-y. Epub 2018 Feb 12. Review. PubMed [citation]PMID: 29435763

Genetic variation in the vitamin D receptor and polycystic ovary syndrome risk. Mahmoudi T. Fertil Steril. 2009 Oct;92(4):1381-3. doi: 10.1016/j.fertnstert.2009.05.002. Epub 2009 Jun 6. PubMed [citation] PMID: 19501823

Green tea prevents non-melanoma skin cancer by enhancing DNA repair. Katiyar SK. Arch Biochem Biophys. 2011 Apr 15;508(2):152-8. doi: 10.1016/j.abb.2010.11.015. Epub 2010 Nov 19. Review. PubMed [citation]PMID: 21094124 PMCID: PMC3077767

Musculoskeletal pain is associated with very low levels of vitamin D in men: results from the European Male Ageing Study. McBeth J, Pye SR, O'Neill TW, Macfarlane GJ, Tajar A, Bartfai G, Boonen S, Bouillon R, Casanueva F, Finn JD, Forti G, Giwercman A, Han TS, Huhtaniemi IT, Kula K, Lean ME, Pendleton N, Punab M, Silman AJ, Vanderschueren D, Wu FC; EMAS Group.. Ann Rheum Dis. 2010 Aug;69(8):1448-52. doi: 10.1136/ard.2009.116053. Epub 2010 May 24. PubMed [citation]PMID: 20498201

New option in photoprotection. Masnec IS, Kotrulja L, Situm M, Poduje S. Coll Antropol. 2010 Apr;34 Suppl 2:257-62. PubMed [citation] PMID: 21302729

Nutrition and melanoma prevention. Jensen JD, Wing GJ, Dellavalle RP. Clin Dermatol. 2010 Nov-Dec;28(6):644-9. doi: 10.1016/j.clindermatol.2010.03.026. Review. PubMed [citation]PMID: 21034988

Polymorphism in vitamin D-binding protein as a genetic risk factor in the pathogenesis of endometriosis. Faserl K, Golderer G, Kremser L, Lindner H, Sarg B, Wildt L, Seeber B. J Clin Endocrinol Metab. 2011 Jan;96(1):E233-41. doi: 10.1210/jc.2010-1532. Epub 2010 Oct 27. PubMed [citation]PMID: 20980430

Serum 25-Hydroxyvitamin D and Bone Mineral Density in a Racially and Ethnically Diverse Group of Men. Hannan MT, Litman HJ, Araujo AB, McLennan CE, McLean RR, McKinlay JB, Chen TC, Holick MF. The Journal of Clinical Endocrinology and Metabolism. 2007 Nov 6; 93(1): 40-46 PMC [article]PMCID: PMC2190744 PMID: 179 86641 DOI: 10.1210/jc.2007-1217

Severe hypocalcemia after intravenous bisphosphonate therapy in occult vitamin D deficiency. Rosen CJ, Brown S. N Engl J Med. 2003 Apr 10;348(15):1503-4. No abstract available. PubMed [citation] PMID: 12686715

The effect of vitamin D replacement therapy on insulin resistance and androgen levels in women with polycystic ovary syndrome. Selimoglu H, Duran C, Kiyici S, Ersoy C, Guclu M, Ozkaya G, Tuncel E, Erturk E, Imamoglu S. J Endocrinol Invest. 2010 Apr;33(4):234-8. doi: 10.3275/6560. Epub 2009 Oct 9. PubMed [citation]PMID: 19820295

The prevalence of headache may be related with the latitude: a possible role of Vitamin D insufficiency? Prakash S, Mehta NC, Dabhi AS, Lakhani O, Khilari M, Shah ND. J Headache Pain. 2010 Aug;11(4):301-7. doi: 10.1007/s10194-010-0223-2. Epub 2010 May 13. Review. PubMed [citation]PMID: 20464624 PMCID: PMC3476351

Ultraviolet B irradiance and incidence rates of bladder cancer in 174 countries. Mohr SB, Garland CF, Gorham ED, Grant WB, Garland FC. Am J Prev Med. 2010 Mar;38(3):296-302. doi: 10.1016/j.amepre.2009.10.044. PubMed [citation]PMID: 20171531

Ultraviolet B irradiance and vitamin D status are inversely associated with incidence rates of pancreatic cancer worldwide. Mohr SB, Garland CF, Gorham ED, Grant WB, Garland FC. Pancreas. 2010 Jul;39(5):669-74. doi: 10.1097/MPA.0b013e3181ce654d. PubMed [citation] PMID: 20442683

Vitamin D and pregnancy: An old problem revisited. Barrett H, McElduff A. Best Pract Res Clin Endocrinol Metab. 2010 Aug;24(4):527-39. doi: 10.1016/j.beem.2010.05.010. Review. PubMed [citation] PMID: 20832734

Vitamin D Beliefs and Associations with Sunburns, Sun Exposure, and Sun Protection. Kim BH, Glanz K, Nehl EJ. International Journal of Environmental Research and Public Health. 2012 Jul 4; 9(7): 2386-2395 PMC [article]PMCID: PMC3407911 PMID: 22851950 DOI: 1 0.3390/ijerph9072386

Vitamin D for cancer prevention: global perspective. Garland CF, Gorham ED, Mohr SB, Garland FC. Ann Epidemiol. 2009 Jul;19(7):468-83. doi: 10.1016/j.annepidem.2009.03.021. Review. PubMed [citation] PMID: 19523595

Vitamin D repletion in patients with primary hyperparathyroidism and coexistent vitamin D insufficiency. Grey A, Lucas J, Horne A, Gamble G, Davidson JS, Reid IR. J Clin Endocrinol Metab. 2005 Apr;90(4):2122-6. Epub 2005 Jan 11. PubMed [citation]PMID: 15644400

Vitamin D: Production, Metabolism, and Mechanisms of Action. Bikle D. 2017 Aug 11. In: Feingold KR, Anawalt B, Boyce A, Chrousos G, Dungan K, Grossman A, Hershman JM, Kaltsas G, Koch C, Kopp P, Korbonits M, McLachlan R, Morley JE, New M, Perreault L, Purnell J, Rebar R, Singer F, et al, editors.Endotext [Internet]. South Dartmouth (MA): MDText.com, Inc.; 2000-. PubMed [citation]PMID: 25905172

Vitamin K Supplement Along with Vitamin D and Calcium Reduced Serum Concentration of Undercarboxylated Osteocalcin While Increasing Bone Mineral Density in Korean Postmenopausal Women over Sixty-Years-Old. Je SH, Joo NS, Choi BH, Kim KM, Kim BT, Park SB, Cho DY, Kim KN, Lee DJ. Journal of Korean Medical Science. 2011 Jul 27; 26(8): 1093-1098 PMC [article]PMCID: PMC3154 347 PMID: 21860562 DOI: 10.3346/jkms.2011.26.8.1093

Vitamin K: Double Bonds beyond Coagulation Insights into Differences between Vitamin K1 and K2 in Health and Disease. Halder M, Petsophonsakul P, Akbulut AC, Pavlic A, Bohan F, Anderson E, Maresz K, Kramann R, Schurgers L. International Journal of Molecular Sciences. 2019 Feb 19; 20(4): 896 PMC [article]PMCID: PMC6413124 P MID: 30791399 DOI: 10.3390/ijms20040896

Bibliography collection

Amor KT, Rashid RM, Mirmirani P. Does D matter? The role of vitamin D in hair disorders and hair follicle cycling. Dermatol Online J. 2010 Feb 15;16(2):3. Review. PubMed PMID: 20178699.

Barrett H, McElduff A. Vitamin D and pregnancy: An old problem revisited. Best Pract Res Clin Endocrinol Metab. 2010 Aug;24(4):527-39. doi: 10.1016/j.beem.2010.05.010. Review. PubMed PMID: 20832734. Cited in PMCRelated citations

Bertone-Johnson ER, Chocano-Bedoya PO, Zagarins SE, Micka AE, Ronnenberg AG. Dietary vitamin D intake, 25-hydroxyvitamin D3 levels and premenstrual syndrome in a college-aged population. J Steroid Biochem Mol Biol. 2010 Jul;121(1-2):434-7. doi: 10.1016/j.

jsbmb.2010.03.076. Epub 2010 Apr 14. PubMed PMID: 20398756. Cited in PMCRelated citations

Bertone-Johnson ER, Hankinson SE, Bendich A, Johnson SR, Willett WC, Manson JE. Calcium and vitamin D intake and risk of incident premenstrual syndrome. Arch Intern Med. 2005 Jun 13;165(11):1246-52. PubMed PMID: 15956003.

Bischoff-Ferrari HA, Dawson-Hughes B, Baron JA, Kanis JA, Orav EJ, Staehelin HB, Kiel DP, Burckhardt P, Henschkowski J, Spiegelman D, Li R, Wong JB, Feskanich D, Willett WC. Milk intake and risk of hip fracture in men and women: a meta-analysis of prospective cohort studies. J Bone Miner Res. 2011 Apr;26(4):833-9. doi: 10.1002/jbmr.279. Erratum in: J Bone Miner Res. 2017 Nov;32(11):2319. PubMed PMID: 20949604. Cited in PMCRelated citations

Brookes GB. Vitamin D deficiency and otosclerosis. Otolaryngol Head Neck Surg. 1985 Jun;93(3):313-21. PubMed PMID: 3927224.

Darling AL, Millward DJ, Torgerson DJ, Hewitt CE, Lanham-New SA. Dietary protein and bone health: a systematic review and meta-analysis. Am J Clin Nutr. 2009 Dec;90(6):1674-92. doi: 10.3945/ajcn.2009.27799. Epub 2009 Nov 4. Review. PubMed PMID: 19889822.

Deluca HF, Prahl JM, Plum LA. 1,25-Dihydroxyvitamin D is not responsible for toxicity caused by vitamin D or 25-hydroxyvitamin D. Arch Biochem Biophys. 2011 Jan 15;505(2):226-30. doi: 10.1016/j.abb.2010.10.012. Epub 2010 Oct 18. PubMed PMID: 20965147. Cited in PMCRelated citations

Faserl K, Golderer G, Kremser L, Lindner H, Sarg B, Wildt L, Seeber B. Polymorphism in vitamin D-binding protein as a genetic risk factor in the pathogenesis of endometriosis. J Clin Endocrinol Metab. 2011 Jan;96(1):E233-41. doi: 10.1210/jc.2010-1532. Epub 2010 Oct 27. PubMed PMID: 20980430. Cited in PMCRelated citations

Garland CF, Gorham ED, Mohr SB, Garland FC. Vitamin D for cancer prevention: global perspective. Ann Epidemiol. 2009 Jul;19(7):468-83. doi: 10.1016/j.annepidem.2009.03.021. Review. PubMed PMID: 19523595.

Giovannucci E. Epidemiology of vitamin D and colorectal cancer: casual or causal link? J Steroid Biochem Mol Biol. 2010 Jul;121(1-2):349-54.

doi: 10.1016/j.jsbmb.2010.03.085. Epub 2010 Apr 14. Review. PubMed PMID: 20398758. Cited in PMCRelated citations

Grey A, Lucas J, Horne A, Gamble G, Davidson JS, Reid IR. Vitamin D repletion in patients with primary hyperparathyroidism and coexistent vitamin D insufficiency. J Clin Endocrinol Metab. 2005 Apr;90(4):2122-6. Epub 2005 Jan 11. PubMed PMID: 15644400.

Heaney R, Garland C, Baggerly C, French C and Gorham E. Letter to Veugelers, P.J. and Ekwaru, J.P., A Statistical Error in the Estimation of the Recommended Dietary Allowance for Vitamin D. Nutrients 2014, 6, 4472-4475; doi: 10.3390/nu6104472. Nutrients 2015, 7, 1688-1690; doi: 10.3390/nu7031688

Jensen JD, Wing GJ, Dellavalle RP. Nutrition and melanoma prevention. Clin Dermatol. 2010 Nov-Dec;28(6):644-9. doi: 10.1016/j.clindermatol.2010.03.026. Review. PubMed PMID: 21034988. Cited in PMCRelated citations

Katiyar SK. Green tea prevents non-melanoma skin cancer by enhancing DNA repair. Arch Biochem Biophys. 2011 Apr 15;508(2):152-8. doi: 10.1016/j.abb.2010.11.015. Epub 2010 Nov 19. Review. PubMed PMID: 21094124; PubMed Central PMCID: PMC3077767. Free full textCited in PMCRelated citations

Khajehei M, Abdali K, Parsanezhad ME, Tabatabaee HR. Effect of treatment with dydrogesterone or calcium plus vitamin D on the severity of premenstrual syndrome. Int J Gynaecol Obstet. 2009 May;105(2):158-61. doi: 10.1016/j.ijgo.2009.01.016. Epub 2009 Feb 20. PubMed PMID: 19232611.

Mahmoudi T. Genetic variation in the vitamin D receptor and polycystic ovary syndrome risk. Fertil Steril. 2009 Oct;92(4):1381-3. doi: 10.1016/j.fertnstert.2009.05.002. Epub 2009 Jun 6. PubMed PMID: 19501823.

Masnec IS, Kotrulja L, Situm M, Poduje S. New option in photoprotection. Coll Antropol. 2010 Apr;34 Suppl 2:257-62. PubMed PMID: 21302729.

McBeth J, Pye SR, O'Neill TW, Macfarlane GJ, Tajar A, Bartfai G, Boonen S, Bouillon R, Casanueva F, Finn JD, Forti G, Giwercman A, Han TS, Huhtaniemi IT, Kula K, Lean ME, Pendleton N, Punab M, Silman AJ, Vanderschueren D, Wu FC; EMAS Group..

Musculoskeletal pain is associated with very low levels of vitamin D in men: results from the European Male Ageing Study. Ann Rheum Dis. 2010 Aug;69(8):1448-52. doi: 10.1136/ard.2009.116053. Epub 2010 May 24. PubMed PMID: 20498201. Cited in PMCRelated citations

Michaëlsson K, Wolk A, Langenskiöld S, Basu S, Warensjö Lemming E, Melhus H, Byberg L. Milk intake and risk of mortality and fractures in women and men: cohort studies. BMJ. 2014 Oct 28;349:g6015. doi: 10.1136/bmj.g6015. PubMed PMID: 25352269; PubMed Central PMCID: PMC4212225. Free full textCited in PMCRelated citations

Mohr SB, Garland CF, Gorham ED, Grant WB, Garland FC. Ultraviolet B irradiance and vitamin D status are inversely associated with incidence rates of pancreatic cancer worldwide. Pancreas. 2010 Jul;39(5):669-74. doi: 10.1097/MPA.0b013e3181ce654d. PubMed PMID: 20442683. Cited in PMCRelated citations

Mohr SB, Garland CF, Gorham ED, Grant WB, Garland FC. Ultraviolet B irradiance and incidence rates of bladder cancer in 174 countries. Am J Prev Med. 2010 Mar;38(3):296-302. doi: 10.1016/j.amepre.2009.10.044. PubMed PMID: 20171531.

Peterlik M, Grant WB, Cross HS. Calcium, vitamin D and cancer. Anticancer Res. 2009 Sep;29(9):3687-98. Review. PubMed PMID: 19667166.

Prakash S, Mehta NC, Dabhi AS, Lakhani O, Khilari M, Shah ND. The prevalence of headache may be related with the latitude: a possible role of Vitamin D insufficiency? J Headache Pain. 2010 Aug;11(4):301-7. doi: 10.1007/s10194-010-0223-2. Epub 2010 May 13. Review. PubMed PMID: 20464624; PubMed Central PMCID: PMC3476351. Free full textCited in PMCRelated citations

Raasch BA, Buettner PG, Garbe C. Basal cell carcinoma: histological classification and body-site distribution. Br J Dermatol. 2006 Aug;155(2):401-7. PubMed PMID: 16882181.

Rosen CJ, Brown S. Severe hypocalcemia after intravenous bisphosphonate therapy in occult vitamin D deficiency. N Engl J Med. 2003 Apr 10;348(15):1503-4. PubMed PMID: 12686715.

Selimoglu H, Duran C, Kiyici S, Ersoy C, Guclu M, Ozkaya G, Tuncel E, Erturk E, Imamoglu S. The effect of vitamin D replacement therapy on insulin resistance and androgen levels in women with polycystic ovary syndrome. J Endocrinol Invest. 2010 Apr;33(4):234-8. doi: 10.3275/6560. Epub 2009 Oct 9. PubMed PMID: 19820295.

Thys-Jacobs S. Alleviation of migraines with therapeutic vitamin D and calcium. Headache. 1994 Nov-Dec;34(10):590-2. PubMed PMID: 7843955.

Thys-Jacobs S. Vitamin D and calcium in menstrual migraine. Headache. 1994 Oct;34(9):544-6. PubMed PMID: 8002332.

Trémezaygues L, Reichrath J. From the bench to emerging new clinical concepts: Our present understanding of the importance of the vitamin D endocrine system (VDES) for skin cancer. Dermatoendocrinol. 2011 Jan;3(1):11-7. doi: 10.4161/derm.3.1.14875. PubMed PMID: 21519403; PubMed Central PMCID: PMC3051847. Free full text-Cited in PMCRelated citations

Wehr E, Pilz S, Schweighofer N, Giuliani A, Kopera D, Pieber TR, Obermayer-Pietsch B. Association of hypovitaminosis D with metabolic disturbances in polycystic ovary syndrome. Eur J Endocrinol. 2009 Oct;161(4):575-82. doi: 10.1530/EJE-09-0432. Epub 2009 Jul 23. PubMed PMID: 19628650.

Yang CS, Wang H, Li GX, Yang Z, Guan F, Jin H. Cancer prevention by tea: Evidence from laboratory studies. Pharmacol Res. 2011 Aug;64(2):113-22. doi: 10.1016/j.phrs.2011.03.001. Epub 2011 Mar 21. Review. PubMed PMID: 21397027. Cited in PMCRelated citations

Yildizhan R, Kurdoglu M, Adali E, Kolusari A, Yildizhan B, Sahin HG, Kamaci M. Serum 25-hydroxyvitamin D concentrations in obese and non-obese women with polycystic ovary syndrome. Arch Gynecol Obstet. 2009 Oct;280(4):559-63. doi: 10.1007/s00404-009-0958-7. Epub 2009 Feb 13. PubMed PMID: 19214546.

Websites:

Environmental Working Group

Skin Cancer.org

Parathyroid.com

Reference

Unexplained Muscle and Joint Pain

Garfinkel, Rachel J., et al. "Vitamin D and Its Effects on Articular Cartilage and Osteoarthritis - Rachel J. Garfinkel, Matthew F. Dilisio, Devendra K. Agrawal, 2017." *SAGE Journals*, journals.sagepub.com/doi/10.1177/2325967117711376.

Heidari, Behzad, Heidari, Parham, Tilaki, Karim Hajian. (7 Jun. 2013) *Relationship between Unexplained Arthralgia and Vitamin D Deficiency: a Case Control Study* http://citeseerx.ist.psu.edu/viewdoc/download?doi =10.1.1.895.2577&rep=rep1&type=pdf

Fibromyalgia

Makrani, Atekeh Hadinezhad, et al. "Vitamin D and Fibromyalgia: a Meta-Analysis." *The Korean Journal of Pain*, The Korean Pain Society, Oct. 2017, www.ncbi.nlm.nih.gov/pmc/articles/PMC5665736/.

Yilmaz, Ramazan, et al. "Efficacy of Vitamin D Replacement Therapy on Patients with Chronic Nonspecific Widespread Musculoskeletal Pain with Vitamin D Deficiency." *International Journal of Rheumatic Diseases*, John Wiley & Sons, Ltd (10.1111), 11 Nov. 2016, onlinelibrary.wiley.com /doi/full/10.1111/1756-185X.12960.

Heart Health

Mheid, Ibhar Al, and Arshed A. Quyyumi. "Vitamin D and Cardiovascular Disease." *JACC*, Journal of the American College of Cardiology, 26 June 2017, www.onlinejacc.org/content/70/1/89.

"Vitamin D and Cardiovascular Disease." *Circulation Research*, www.ahajournals.org/doi/10.1161/CIRCRESAHA.113.301241.

Muscogiuri, Giovanna "Vitamin D and cardiovascular disease: From atherosclerosis to myocardial infarction and stroke" *International Journal of Cardiology* March 1, 2017 Volume 230, Pages 577–584

https://www.internationaljournalofcardiology.com/article/
S0167-5273(16)34541-7/abstract

S, A., & Mehta V. (2017, February 17). Does Vitamin D Deficiency Lead to Hypertension? Retrieved from https://www.cureus.com/articles/6257-does-vitamin-d-deficiency-lead-to-hypertension

Mehta, V., & Agarwal, S. (2017, February 17). Does Vitamin D Deficiency Lead to Hypertension? Retrieved from https://www.ncbi.nlm.nih.gov/pmc/articles/PMC5356990/

Vitamin D and Cardiovascular Disease: Controversy Unresolved. (2017, June 26). Retrieved from https://www.sciencedirect.com/science/article/pii/S0735109717374843

Hypothyroidism

Effect of Vitamin D deficiency treatment on thyroid ... (n.d.). Retrieved from http://jrms.mui.ac.ir/files/journals/1/articles/10696/public/10696-39904-1-PB.pdf

Idiculla J, Prabhu P, Pradeep R, Khadilkar K, Kannan S. Vitamin D and primary hypothyroidism: Is there an association?. Thyroid Res Pract [serial online] 2018 [cited 2019 May 13];15:34-7. Available from: http://www.thetrp.net/text.asp?2018/15/1/34/228382

Vahabi Anaraki, P., Aminorroaya, A., Amini, M., Momeni, F., Feizi, A., Iraj, B., & Tabatabaei, A. (2017, September 26). Effect of Vitamin D deficiency treatment on thyroid function and autoimmunity markers in Hashimoto's thyroiditis: A double-blind randomized placebo-controlled clinical trial. Retrieved from https://www.ncbi.nlm.nih.gov/pmc/articles/PMC5629831/

Vitamin D, Autoimmunity and Your Thyroid. (2018, July 26). Retrieved from https://www.wilsonssyndrome.com/vitamin-d-thyroid/

(PDF) Vitamin D and primary hypothyroidism: Is there an ... (n.d.). Retrieved from https://www.researchgate.net/publication/323962284_Vitamin_D_and_primary_hypothyroidism_Is_there_an_association

Migraines

Tayebeh Mottaghi, Fariborz Khorvash, Gholamreza Askari, Mohammad Reza Maracy, Reza Ghiasvand, Zahra Maghsoudi, Bijan Iraj

J Res Med Sci. 2013 Mar; 18(Suppl 1): S66–S70.

Tae-Jin Song, Min-Kyung Chu, Jong-Hee Sohn, Hong-Yup Ahn, Sun Hwa Lee, Soo-Jin Cho

J Clin Neurol. 2018 Jul; 14(3): 366–373. Published online 2018 Jun 29. doi: 10.3988/jcn.2018.14.3.366 PMCID: PMC6031995

Mottaghi, Tayebeh, et al. "The Relationship between Serum Levels of Vitamin D and Migraine." *Journal of Research in Medical Sciences : the Official Journal of Isfahan University of Medical Sciences*, Medknow Publications & Media Pvt Ltd, Mar. 2013, www.ncbi.nlm.nih.gov/pubmed/23961291.

Song, Tae Jin, et al. "Effect of Vitamin D Deficiency on the Frequency of Headaches in Migraine." *Journal of Clinical Neurology (Seoul, Korea)*, Korean Neurological Association, July 2018, www.ncbi.nlm.nih.gov/pmc/articles/PMC6031995/.

Infertility and Ovulation

Lata, I., Tiwari, S., Gupta, A., Yadav, S., & Yadav, S. (2017). To Study the Vitamin D Levels in Infertile Females and Correlation of Vitamin D Deficiency with AMH Levels in Comparison to Fertile Females. Retrieved from https://www.ncbi.nlm.nih.gov/pmc/articles/PMC5586095/ (To Study the Vitamin D Levels in Infertile Females and Correlation of Vitamin D Deficiency with AMH Levels in Comparison to Fertile Females)

Soares, J. B., Beck, R. T., Neto, T. B., Carbonar, M. B., Moreira, L., & Okamoto, C. T. (2018, February 08). Vitamin D: An effect on fertility and in vitro fertilization. Retrieved from http://humanreproductionarchives.com/article/doi/10.4322/hra.001517

Depression

Cuomo, Giordano, N., Goracci, A., & Fagiolini, A. (n.d.). Depression and Vitamin D Deficiency: Causality, Assessment, and Clinical Practice Implications. Retrieved from http://www.jneuropsychiatry.org/peer-review/depression-and-vitamin-d-deficiency-causality-assessment-and-clinical-practice-implications-12051.html

High Dose Vitamin D Supplementation Is Associated With a Reduction in Depression Score Among Adolescent Girls: A Nine-Week Follow-Up

Study. (n.d.). Retrieved from https://www.tandfonline.com/doi/abs/ 10.1080/19390211.2017.1334736

Journal of Affective Disorders. (n.d.). (2017 January 15). Volume 208. P. 56-61 Retrieved from https://www.sciencedirect.com/journal/journal -of-affective-disorders/vol/208/suppl/C

Disorders

Vitamin D and depression. (2016, October 11). Retrieved from https:// www.sciencedirect.com/science/article/pii/S0165032716308928

Anxiety

Martino, G., Catalano, A., Bellone, F., Sardella, A., Lasco, C., Caprì, T., . . . Morabito, N. (n.d.). Vitamin D status is associated with anxiety levels in postmenopausal women evaluated for osteoporosis. Retrieved from http://cab.unime.it/journals/index.php/MJCP/article/view/1740

Vazquez, M., Ortiz, N., Martínez, V., Roman, L., Bauman, K., Melo, M., . . . Colman, I. A. (2018, June 01). AB0599 Relation between the deficit/deficiency of vitamin d and the depression/anxiety in patients with lupus in the department of rheumatology of the hospital of clinics. Retrieved from https://ard.bmj.com/content/77/Suppl_2/1451.1

Psychosis

J. Lally, P. Gardner-Sood, M. Firdosi, C. Iyegbe, B. Stubbs, K. Green-wood, . . . F. Gaughran. (2016, March 22). Clinical correlates of vita-min D deficiency in established psychosis. Retrieved from https:// bmcpsychiatry.biomedcentral.com/articles/10.1186/s12888-016-0780-2

Miller, B., MD,PhD, MPH. (n.d.). Cognitive Disorders | Psychiatric Times. Retrieved from https://www.psychiatrictimes.com/cognitive-disorders

Insomnia

Han, Bin; Zhu, Fu-Xiang; Shi, Chao; Wu, Heng-Lan; Gu, Xiao-Hong. 2017. "Association between Serum Vitamin D Levels and Sleep Distur-bance in Hemodialysis Patients." *Nutrients* 9, no. 2: 139.

Body Weight

Mason C, Xiao L, Imayama I, Duggan C, Wang C-Y, Korde L, McTiernan A. Vitamin D3supplementation during weight loss: a double-blind randomized controlled trial. Am J Clin Nutr 2014;99:1015–25. Erratum. (2014, October 01). Retrieved from https://academic.oup.com/ajcn/article/100/4/1213/4576597

Mason, C., Xiao, L., Imayama, I., Duggan, C., Wang, C., Korde, L., & McTiernan, A. (2014, May). Vitamin D3 supplementation during weight loss: A double-blind randomized controlled trial. Retrieved from https://www.ncbi.nlm.nih.gov/pmc/articles/PMC3985208/

The Impact of Vitamin D on Weight Loss – touchENDOCRINOLOGY. (2014, February 03). Retrieved from https://www.touchendocrinology.com/the-impact-of-vitamin-d-on-weight-loss/

Obesity

The Convergence of Two Epidemics: Vitamin D Deficiency in Obese School-aged Children. (2017, October 18). Retrieved from https://www.sciencedirect.com/science/article/pii/S0882596316304298

Trends to Promote a More Proatherogenic Cardiometabolic ... (n.d.). Retrieved from http://journals.sagepub.com/doi/abs/10.1177/0003319714528569

Vanlint, S. (2013, March 20). Vitamin D and obesity. Retrieved from https://www.ncbi.nlm.nih.gov/pmc/articles/PMC3705328/

Inflammatory Bowel Disease

Ardesia, Marco, Guido Ferlazzo, and Walter Fries. "Vitamin D and Inflammatory Bowel Disease." BioMed Research International. 2015. Accessed May 13, 2019. https://www.ncbi.nlm.nih.gov/pmc/articles/PMC4427008/.

Caviezel, Daniel, Silvia Maissen, Hendrik Niess, Caroline Kiss, and Petr Hruz. "High Prevalence of Vitamin D Deficiency among Patients with Inflammatory Bowel Disease." Inflammatory Intestinal Diseases. June 28, 2018. Accessed May 13, 2019. https://www.karger.com/Article/FullText/489010.

"P131 VITAMIN D DEFICIENCY MAY BE ASSOCIATED WITH ..." Accessed May 13, 2019. https://www.gastrojournal.org/article/S0016-5085(17)36535-6/fulltext.

Diabetes and Insulin Resistance

Gao, Yun, Zheng, Xingwu, Ren, Yan, Chen, Tao, Zhong, Li, Yan, Donge, Yan, Wu, Tian, and Haoming. "Vitamin D and Incidence of Prediabetes or Type 2 Diabetes: A Four-Year Follow-Up Community-Based Study." Disease Markers. March 18, 2018. Accessed May 13, 2019. https://www.hindawi.com/journals/dm/2018/1926308/. :The current prospective study suggests that low 25(OH)D levels might have contributed to the incidence of prediabetes or T2DM in Chinese individuals.

Psoriasis

Barrea, Luigi, Maria Cristina Savanelli, Carolina Di Somma, Maddalena Napolitano, Matteo Megna, Annamaria Colao, and Silvia Savastano. "Vitamin D and Its Role in Psoriasis: An Overview of the Dermatologist and Nutritionist." SpringerLink. February 07, 2017. Accessed May 13, 2019. https://link.springer.com/article/10.1007/s11154-017-9411-6.

Venegas-Iribarren, Soledad, and Romina Andino. "Topical Corticosteroids or Vitamin D Analogues for Plaque Psoriasis?" Medwave. June 27, 2017. Accessed May 13, 2019. https://www.ncbi.nlm.nih.gov/pubmed/28665918.

Eczema

Jung Kim, Soo-Nyung Kim, Yang Won Lee, Yong Beom Choe, and Kyu Joong Ahn. "Vitamin D Status and Efficacy of Vitamin D Supplementation in Atopic Dermatitis: A Systematic Review and Meta-Analysis." MDPI. December 03, 2016. Accessed May 13, 2019. https://www.mdpi.com/2072-6643/8/12/789.

Palmer, Debra J. "Vitamin D and the Development of Atopic Eczema." MDPI. May 20, 2015. Accessed May 13, 2019. https://www.mdpi.com/2077-0383/4/5/1036.

Digestive Disorders

Khayyat, Yasir, and Suzan Attar. "Vitamin D Deficiency in Patients with Irritable Bowel Syndrome: Does It Exist?" Oman Medical Journal. March 2015. Accessed May 13, 2019. https://www.ncbi.nlm.nih.gov/pmc/articles/PMC4412886/.

Williams, Claire E., Elizabeth A. Williams, and Bernard M. Corfe. "Vitamin D Status in Irritable Bowel Syndrome and the Impact of Supplementation on Symptoms: What Do We Know and What Do We Need to Know?" Nature News. January 25, 2018. Accessed May 13, 2019. https://www.nature.com/articles/s41430-017-0064-z#article-info.

Index

About the Author

LANI SIMPSON, DC, CCD, is a chiropractic doctor and a Certified Clinical (bone) Densitometrist (CCD). She has been a leading expert in integrative medicine for over 30 years. Dr. Simpson is the author of the highly acclaimed book, *Dr. Lani's No Nonsense Bone Health Guide* and the National PBS show, *Stronger Bones Longer Life*.

Dr. Simpson's new book, *Dr. Lani's No-Nonsense Sun Health Guide* was inspired by her experience with over 20 skin cancer diagnoses due to frequent early childhood sunburns. And, although she lived in "sunny California" in her forties, she was diagnosed with a vitamin D deficiency and osteoporosis. These diagnoses led her to unravel the healing nature of the sun through being mindful that too much sun can be harmful. Her journey led her to understand safe sun exposure, sun-induced vitamin D production, vitamin D supplementation, and safe sunscreen products for the whole family. She is passionate about teaching others to engage with the sun while reaping the healing benefits and avoiding skin damage.